THE MOOR
NATURES HEALING MIRACLE

The Moor

Natures Healing Miracle

for

Health - Rejuvination - Beauty

PETER J. HUDSON

MAYFAIR PUBLISHING

Disclaimer

The information in this book cannot and is not intended to replace the skills of a physician. Neither the publisher or author may be held responsible for any damage direct or indirect that may be caused following any of the treatments in this book.

© Peter John Hudson 1993

Mayfair Publishing
PO Box 860
Eastbourne
East Sussex, BN20 7DJ
United Kingdom

British Library catalogueing-in-publication data.
ISBN 1-898572-00-3

Cover Illustration by Elizabeth Jenks
Typesetting and printing on recycled
paper by Ashprint, Eastbourne
Bound by Kensett Ltd., Hove

No part of this book may be reproduced in any form without permission in writing from the copyright owners, except by a reviewer, who is welcome to quote brief passages.

Foreword

With gratitude and pleasure I have received the request from my good friend, Peter Hudson, to write a foreword for a book on treatments originating from *The Neydharting Moor* in Austria. This Austrian moor has long been recognised universally for its famous positive therapeutic effects. For over thirty years I have been familiar with the wide range of holistic health treatments obtained from these sources and many of my patients will bear witness to their gentle efficacy.

When, in the late Fifties, together with the well-known naturopathic Swiss doctor, Alfred Vogel, I opened the very first clinic of natural cures in The Netherlands, we made a conscious decision. At that time Dr. Vogel insisted that special arrangements be made for different forms of treatment which incorporated the *Neydharting Moor* methods. He went so far as to arrange visits for me to German and Swiss clinics so that I could see these therapies put to use first hand. At some of the institutes visited I witnessed encouraging successes achieved when these treatment methods were used for specific ailments, but also for general health maintenance. It has always been a disappointment to me that so few people were then aware of the healing purposes of *Neydharting Moor* treatments.

Fortunately, the popularity of Neydharting Moor therapies is steadily increasing. This does not surprise me as over the years I have seen the gentle, beneficial and effective results of these methods and I can wholeheartedly support the gratitude of the many patients who have undergone *Neydharting Moor* treatment methods.

It was essential, and not before time, that a book was written on the various ways and methods originating from Neydharting Moor could be used for a wider populace and the publishers could not have done better than approaching my good friend, Peter Hudson. I have known Peter as a friend and a colleague for many years. There is absolutely no question as to Peter's belief and faith in, and commitment to, natural cures. He is fortunate in that his family fully supports him in his work and beliefs, and has done so for many years. He not only preaches natural treatments, but successfully puts them into practice for himself and many others. His total commitment is the strength of Peter's success and during his years as a practitioner he has been instrumental in providing comfort to many of his patients.

This time, through the book, he is hoping to reach many more people and it is my sincere wish that he will be successful in informing people of the beneficial effects of the Neydharting Moor methods in the treatment of specific ailments, and educating them in their usefulness for general health maintenance. From the very first chapter one gets engrosed in what can only be called "common sense". At all times Peter credits Nature for its good counselling the force of Nature will be able to deal with what mankind has caused to become unbalanced.

Hence, my grateful thanks for being invited to write the foreword for this excellent book and my sincerest wish that Peter's message on the beneficial methods based on the natural therapies and healing abilities originating from the Neydharting Moor of Austria are well received.

>   Jan de Vries
>   Auchenkyle, Southwoods
>   Troon, Scotland

Acknowledgments

During the preparation of this book I have been much indebted to Diane Ash for her painstaking and patient typing. To Peter and Dee Unruh, Directors of Austrian Moor Life UK; Rupert Ashford and Zoe Hamlyn for their skill and invaluable assistance in design and production; Elizabeth Jenks for artwork; Nigel Garion-Hutchings for Kirlian photography; but most of all to Professor Otto Stober, founder of the Neydharting Moor Health Clinic, Austria and the many scientists, doctors and researchers at the Austrian Moor Research Institute whose dedication and work has made this book possible. My special thanks to Jan de Vries for writing the foreword to this book.

Finally to my wife Yvonne for her help, patience and understanding.

Contents

Foreward	v
Acknowledgements	vii
Preface	xii
Introduction	xiii
The Neydharting Moor of Austria	1
Herbs of the Moor and their Indications	7
Quinta Essentia	21
Taking the Healing Waters	27
The Moor for Natural Beauty	41
Healing And Cleansing	47
Head to Toe Health and Beauty - The Moor Way	51
Moor, an Elixir of Youth	55
Moor Life for Women	59
The Moor for Sportsmen and Women	65

Colon Health	67
Moor Life Massage	73
Hair - Scalp - Dental - Hand Care	79
Animals - Pets - Plants - Garden	83
Life Energy Fields	91
Scientific and Medical Opinions including Reports	95
Cases from the Authors Practice	119
Healing Reactions	135
Dietetic Considerations	137
Authors Personal Testimony	141
In Perfect Harmony with Nature	143
The Moor Song	145
Conclusion	146
Austrian Moor UK Practioners Association	147
Austrian Moor Life UK	148
The Author	149

Clinics who use the Neydharting Moor	150
Glossary	152
References	155
Index	157
Notes	

Preface

The Neydharting Moor of Austria is famous for its holistic health treatments which have very positive therapeutic effects. Satisfied users state that the healing action of the various Moor treatments have helped them overcome a host of different ailments ranging from inflammatory conditions of the joints and muscles, circulatory complaints, hormonal and female problems, gastro-intestinal and skin troubles, ulcers and auto-immune deficiency diseases, to name but a few.

No wonder the Moor at Neydharting has been known throughout history as miraculous in its healing abilities. Whilst the Neydharting Moor treatments are rapidly increasing in popularity, many people lack awareness of the proper role in both the treatment of specific ailments and health maintenance.

It is my sincere hope that this book will be considered a comprehensive guide to the subject of using the Moor for maximum therapeutic efficacy. You will learn how the Moor can correct all manner of health problems by giving to the organism exactly what it requires thus assisting the body to heal itself.

As a holistic and natural medicine practitioner of at least 35 years in active practice, I consider the Moor Health Treatments perhaps the safest and most effective way of overcoming a whole diversity of tenacious health problems.

Introduction

In order to understand more fully the material in this book, it will be helpful to the reader if he or she knows a little about the relationship between the cells and nutrition.

The body is composed of trillions of tiny electrically charged cells of various kinds, for example blood cells, nerve cells, bone cells, brain cells, organ and gland cells. These cells are all closely bonded together in differing groups, thus forming the many tissues, organs and structures that make up the human body. The number and type of cells in various groups, also the way in which they are bonded together, decides the resultant form and functioning of each tissue that makes up the organs and various structures. All the cells are immersed in and entirely surrounded by a fluid called intercellular fluid. This fluid is a living ocean containing all the various nutrients which are required for healthy functioning.

The systems growth, heat and energy, and repair are all dependant upon the correct nutrition of the trillions of cells of which it is constructed. Should there be a deficiency of the various nutrients required, or if the intercellular spaces become cluttered with toxic waste matter so that oxygen cannot reach the cells, cell function is seriously impaired, thus resulting in various manifestations of illness.

The continuous changes occurring in the cells is known as cell metabolism, this consists of the building up of cell structure known as anabolism. These most vital chemical changes give rise to heat and energy. Correct cell metabolism depends on an adequate supply of oxygen, water, and vital nutrients and an unhampered freedom of circulation of blood the very medium in which oxygen, water and nutrients are carried to the cells.

Therefore freedom of this most important process is dependant upon a free flowing circulation which results from the right type of muscular movement and exercise. All the trillions of cells which make up our very being are nourished by the food we eat. Water too is essential in order to maintain the blood's normal water requirements.

For many thousands of years man has evolved and thrived upon natural foods including herbs. Then approximately fifty or more years ago various methods of food refining were developed, the result being white flour and other devitalised grains, also sugar, all these deprived of their vital nutrients. The consumption of these refined and adulterated foods, if you can call them such, has increased to massive proportions resulting in many forms of ill health to the consumer. The above products and those derived from them are highly acid forming and act as a systematic poison to the human body.

Add to the above all the other thousands of manufactured foodstuffs mass-produced in factories. They are all canned, bottled, packeted rubbish, useless as proper nourishment to the body, they are dead foods which can only in the long run destroy our health and vitality, thus shortening our lives.

The health of the nation has been put at risk by the producers of these dead foods, as also by the manufacturers of chemical substances used both in foods, and on the land for the growing of crops.

Little wonder that the body breaks down and dies long before its allotted span of time. Given the right foods, along with herbs and the right environment, the body is a self-regulating and self-healing organism capable of putting right its own troubles, however, sometimes it requires assistance.It must be remembered that all symptoms of ill health are only an outward sign of internal disorder; they are the means whereby the body draws attention to itself and asks for help.

It is not an exaggeration to say that so long as cell nutrition and cell respiration is adequate the system is practically immune from disease. With a clean bloodstream containing all the vital nutrients disease would have a difficult task in taking hold.

As a natural medicine practitioner and as is expected from that perspective, I have dedicated over thirty years in the search for health amongst the World of Nature. I believe that a disease can only be cured naturally by man's own inherent healing powers and the assistance from physicians.

We should stop and reflect upon the marvellous vitality of the earth which expresses itself most profoundly in the ceaseless cycle of the green leaf of the trees, shrubs, plants, grasses and herbs. Every year trees, shrubs, plants, grasses and herbs have returned their vital force even in the dormant stage. During spring small buds which quickly develop in to green leaves rich in chlorophyll and other nutrients become darker in colour and develop as a result of receiving vital energy from the sun, dews, rains and nutrients from the earth.

When spring and early summer arrives it is a most wonderful experience to witness the fields, mountains, forests, woodlands, meadows and moorlands again covered with green. As the leaves on the trees and plants, we are refreshed and regain our vigour; this the poets know, however, is the sight of green so insignificant as to be confined only to the psyche of man? I cannot but think that present day man has overlooked the power of nature in favour of modern science and technology.

If it was not for an abundance of green grasses, trees and herbs in this world, very few creatures including man himself could possibly survive for long. Herbs especially were given to the animals and mankind by an all wise Creature Intelligence and according to Biblical records the herbs of the fields were among the foods chosen by the Creator as a necessary part of man and animals diet at the dawn of history.

In this modern scientific and technological age man is inclined to ignore these natural healing and health maintaining foods and instead reach out for the latest wonder drugs which more often than not produce undesirable toxic side effects which are even worse than the actual illness for which they are prescribed. It is a sorry fact that a good twenty five per cent of hospital admissions are due to the side effects of allopathic drug medication. Also, even more disturbing, very many people die as a result from the long term effects of such drugs.

I would like to see all medical practitioners teach their patients that only Nature is the Healer. Disease after all is the restorative powers of nature to eliminate from the diseased organism the various conditions responsible for the illness in the first place. All diseases, no matter what symptoms they exhibit are a violation in one way or another of nature's constructive laws and principles.

In times of illness our bodies should be given every assistance in its self healing efforts to expel the disease producing toxins and poisons. Providing we use natural means when ill the organism will in time heal itself for the body is self-repairing, self-rejuvenating and self-building. Like the creatures of the wilds we also possess an innate healing intelligence.

Herbs are possibly the most potent of all plants, the majority are the same now as they were all those millions of years ago. Herbs, leaves, seeds, barks and roots contain a vital force as well as specific chemical agents, they are dissolvers, openers of obstructions, eliminators of dead elements and waste materials; they cleanse and purify the whole organism. Any inflammation, infection or putrification is resisted by their various therapeutic agents. They are an antidote to poisons and toxins and a natural relief from aches and pains.

Herbal elements in a combined and synergistic form as nature intended normalise the body chemistry and metabolism thus acting as a tonic to the numerous psycho-physiological functions of the whole system.

The Neydharting Moor consists of a wealth of organic constituents from hundreds of different herbs that come in a form easily and readily absorbable by the millions of cells in the body either taken internally or applied externally.

Although herbs are slow workers they carry out their healing action deeply and thoroughly without dangerous side effects. For this reason and without any reservation I recommend the Neydharting Moor Health Treatments. Furthermore they are unique compared with other herbal agents in that they contain not just one or two herbal ingredients but the many active biological, bio-mineral and organic substances derived over thousands of years from hundreds of medicinal herbs, plants, roots, stalks, blooms, fruits, seeds, leaves and tubers which have been known for centuries in folk medicine. Their healing efficacy have stood the test of time, proof of which is in the amazing cures as witnessed by very many physicians interested in the curative effects of the Neydharting Moor.

Over many years I have had the privilege of recommending to my patients the various Moor range of health and beauty treatments which have in many cases produced complete reversals of chronic ill health and a remarkable slowing down of the biological ageing process resulting in rejuvenation of the whole body.

This book will in addition to the various many indications and applications of the Moor treatments summarize most interesting medical research carried out by Moor Scientists. Should you decide to try the Moors Healing Waters it is my sincere hope that your experiences of the Moor in its various holistic healing forms will be your first step on a journey towards health and wellbeing.

Peter J Hudson

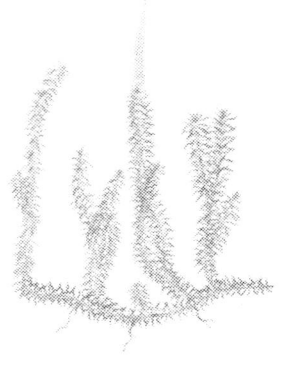

Dedicated to Professor O Stober
1902 - 1990

When Professor Otto Stober first visited the Neydharting Moor in 1939 he sensed the whole area was of particular importance. Then began months of intensive research in the local library and listening to the local villagers who had incredible stories to tell about the Neydharting Valley and its precious Moor.

A year later Professor Otto Stober decided to invest into what is now a part of history. He bought the Neydharting 130 acre site in 1940 when it then contained an 8 bedroomed Clinic. 53 years later it is now a 400 bedroom Clinic with a 2 year waiting list, with the Neydharting Moor being freely prescribed on the Medical Aid Schemes (equivalent to our NHS) of Austria, Germany, Switzerland, Italy and France.

Many superlatives have been attributed to Professor Otto Stober throughout his life, but mankind owes him the greatest debt of all. For without his vision, research, enthusiasm and dedication, the world would have missed one of Natures truely greatest treasures.

We dedicate this book to his memory.

Peter David Unruh
Managing Director
AUSTRIAN MOOR PRODUCTS LTD

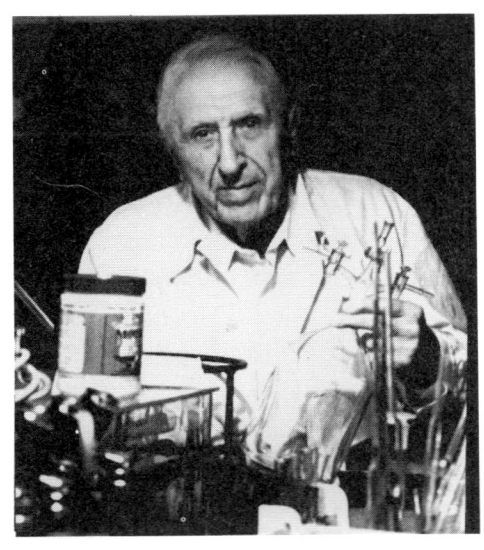

Important Dates re Professor Stober

1945 : Start of the building of the Neydharting Clinic which Professor Stober totally designed himself.

1948 : Honourable member of the International Medical Academy of Rome, Italy.

1951 : Founded the International Moor Museum officially classified as an historical monument.

1952 : The first International Congress for Research on Moor in Salzburg and now held every 18 months in Austria and attended by Moor Research Scientists and Doctors throughout Europe.

1954 : Founder and honoured president of the International research on the Moor.

1956 : Founder member of the International Society of Paracelsus in Salzburg.

1962 : Silver Medal from the Chamber of Commerce, Upper Austria.
1970 : President of Austria awards the title 'Professor' to Otto Stober.
1981 : Austrian Government awards the Clinic the use of the National Coat of Arms of the Republic of Austria.

The Neydharting Moor of Austria

The Moor at Neydharting is older than the Bible, it is situated in a unique lowland moor in upper Austria approximately sixty kilometres from Salzburg.

From early as 800 B.C. the Moor has been used in times of illness and injury by humans and animals alike. It has been recorded that the first to discover the healing and curative effects of the Moor were the Celts. Excavations have revealed ancient Celtic wooden huts which had been preserved in the Moor.

Old hunting chronicles and the observation of wild creatures suggest that injured and sick animals sought out the healing qualities of the Moor waters. Poisoned dogs and cats would drag themselves long distances to take the waters and more often than not were cured.

Paracelsus, the famous alchemist and physician stayed at Neydharting Moor in the 16th century. He believed he had discovered in the Moor the "Quinta Essentia", The Remedy. The Neydharting Health Spa has to this day been visited by many thousands of people from all parts of Europe. Amongst its famous patrons have been Louis XIV and Napoleon and Josephine, also many of the Nobility from Europe.

Scientists at the early part of the 20th century conducted tests to find the chemical agents responsible for the Moors remarkable healing abilities experienced by generations. To this present day investigation and scientific research continues on the Moor to determine exactly how its healing effects occur, as a result of this research there is available a plethora of medical evidence proving its impact and therapeutic efficacy in all manner of diseases.

Over the last 40 or more years some 500 leading scientists and Doctors from Europe have clinically tested the Moor. Their findings have made it possible to offer medical treatment for a whole range of conditions which is recognised and recommended by the National Medical Insurance Schemes of Austria, Germany, Italy, Switzerland and France where it has remained a leader of natural treatment for a whole diversity of chronic illnesses over the last 30 years or so.

A greater part of the Moor research work was undertaken by Professor O. Stober who carried it out in an untiring and dedicated manner from 1942 to his passing in 1990 The Neydharting Health Spa including many thousands of grateful patients and users the world over of the Moor health products are indebted to him for producing such a unique and highly efficacious range of health treatments.

It may interest the reader to know that 400 patients can be accommodated at Neydharting at any one time, the majority of patients staying from 10 to 21 days undertaking the famous Moor treatments. The Spa is fully booked up for 2 years in advance. This in itself is evidence of the remarkable healing powers of the Moor.

The Neydharting Moor is unique compared with other moors simply because not all mud deposits consist of healing factors. The moors that have beneficial healing effects are known as pelloids. They are uncommon and are only found providing certain necessary biological and geological factors are present which bring into existence the ideal conditions for a healing moor. The Moor consists mainly of organic pelloids brought about over many thousands of years through the gradual decomposition of hundreds of plants and herbs resulting in exceptional healing properties due mainly to the high concentration of rich organic elements.

Furthermore the Neydharting Moor is the only known moor in Europe, possibly the World, which to this day has retained all of its organic abundance resulting in quite spectacular healing properties. Due to its geographical location in the Neydharting Valley Basin the waters have never drained away, also the Moor has not dried out over the years therefore retaining all of its natural organic, mineral and trace element factors. In comparison the majority of other moors have at some time during their existence completely dried out resulting in the total loss of their organic substances.

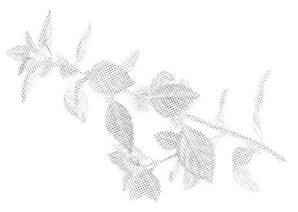

For the reader to fully comprehend what is Moor it is necessary to know the meaning of the word. I could do no better than quote Professor O. Stober ''Moor does not mean simply moor''. The Austrian Moor Research Institute and the International Association for Moor Research regards peat as an end product derived from the decomposition of rotting trees which have been in submersion of water for a considerable period of time. Owing to the absence of oxygen the trees undergo decay through putrefaction which causes certain chemical changes to take place resulting in cellulose; taking into consideration that trees consist mainly of cellulose all that is left is further cellulose.

On the other hand the Moor at Neydharting is the result of interacting chemicals, biological and bio-chemical changes which are reliant upon flora and fauna being present including a favourable climatic and geological environment. A further important pre-requisite for a medicinal moor is that it must have evolved from hundreds of herbal species and plants in their entirety, i.e., roots, stalks, blooms, fruits, seeds, tubers and leaves which the Neydharting Moor originates from.

The wide range of therapeutic properties present in the living herbs and plants such as vitamins, minerals, trace and micro agents, hormones and antibiotics are all held and preserved in the final stages of the process. This unique molecular structure is present in all of the Moor treatments and as Moor is merely harvested and not manufactured or given any chemical preservatives etc. it can be truly said that it is "The Living Gift of Nature" which modern science cannot come even close to.

Quite some unusual sightings can be observed at the Moor. Weeping Willow trees, instead of their branches hanging and spreading downwards, grow upwards towards the sky and heavens. Locals refer to them as "Laughing Willows" In winter when all round the temperature drops to many degrees below sub-zero, the Moor never freezes. It will be of interest to note that during the Chernobyl disaster when a radioactive cloud passed overhead, tests on the Moor carried out by scientists revealed that it was unaffected. One can experience whilst walking round the Moor first thing in the morning and late at night a peace and silence which is quite ethereal.

Many creatures including birds who live in and around the Neydharting Moor cannot be found anywhere else in the world, also fish, frogs and newts are much larger than is normal and display extraordinary colours. Dead bodies of animals dug from the Moor believed to be thousands of years old are completely preserved including the soft substance of their brains. Apples and other fruit if put into the Moor remains fresh for a much longer period, likewise eggs placed in the Moor do not go rotten.

Finally, the Moor has won official approval from the Austrian Government. Over the past twenty years there have been nine International Scientific Congresses on Universal Moor Research attended by eminent representatives of the medical world who concluded that the Neydharting Moor is the only known medicinal moor of therapeutic worth.

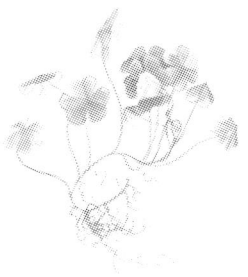

"All medicine is in the earth"
(Paracelsus)

Herbs of the Moor and their Indications

The following list of herbs from the Neydharting Moor and their therapeutic indications have been taken from Dr. Wolfgang Paul D.Sc. Book, Healing Earth Moor

English & Scientific Terms	Indications
Devil's bit (Succisa Pratensis)	*Heavy breathing*
Pearl-wort	*Urinary complaint*
Elecampane (Inula Helenium)	*Haemorrhoids*
Horehound (Marrubium)	*Intestinal catarrh*
Wood angelica 9angelica Silvestris)	*Wounds*
Fetid chara or stonewort (Chara Fetida)	*Glands*
Arnica (Arnica Montana)	*Bleedings*
Dwarf-elder-root (Sambucus Ebulus) (Ebulum Humile)	*Urinary bleeding*
Eyebright, euphrasy (Euphrasia)	*Weak sight*
Brooklime (Veronica Beccabunga)	*Conjunctiva*
Bennet, avens (Geum/Urbanum)	*Gums*
Badekraut	*Intestinal complaint*
Valerian (Valeriana Officinalis)	*Heart*
Bear's bilberry (Arcto-staphylos Uva Ursi)	*Disease of the kidneys*
Club-moss (Moor Powder) (Lycopodium) or enchanter's nightshade (Circaea)	*Liver complaint*
Barlauch	*Arteriosclerosis*
Common or sweet basil (Ocymum Basilicum)	*Stone in the bladder; cystic calculus*
Mugwort (Artemisia)	*Epilepsy*
Bog-asphodel (Narthecium Ossifragum)	*Injuries to the bones*
Comfrey (Symphytum)	*Fracture of a bone*
Common broom (Sarothamnus or Cystisus Scoparius)	*Flatulency*
Henbane, hog's bean (Hyoscyamus Niger)	*Arthritis*
Rush, moss rush, heath rush, (Iuncus Squarrosus)	*Rash; eruptions on the skin*

Herbs of the Moor awnd their Indications

Bindengwachse	Fatty degeneration
Birches, moor birches (Betula)	Hair disease
Common buck-bean	Blood deficiency; anaemia
Cuckoo-flower (Cardamine Pratensis)	Mucosa
Flowering Rush (Butomus Umbellatus)	Diarrhoea
Finger-fern (Comarum Palustre)	Women's disease
Blood-wort (or dock)	
Potentilla Tormentilla)	Diarrhoea
Purple loosestrife (Lythrum Salicarica)	Kidney
Fenugreek	Abscesses
Brownwort (Scrophularia)	Scrofulosis
Brennkraut	Eczema
Bramble	Intestine
Bruesch	Uterus
Water-cress (Nasturtium/Officinale)	Urine
Water moss	Venereal disease
Butter-flower, marigold	Pimples, blotches; acne
Marsh-mallow root	Cough
Aconite (Aconitum)	Trigeminal neuralgia
Iron wort, vervain	Wounds
Gentian (Gentiana)	Stomach
Strawberry plant (Fragaria)	Fall of the hair, alopecia
Fumitory (Fumaria)	(Eyes)
Alder-bush	Wounds
Black alder (Frangula almus)	(Laxative)
Dyer's weed	Gall bladder
Fennel (Foeniculum)	Bladder-ailment
Butterwort (Pinguicula)	Lungs
Marsh trefoil, bogbean	
(Menyanthes Trifoliata)	Fever
Soft rush (Iuncas Effusus)	Stomach
Fletchbinse	Dysentery
Carnivorous fly-orchis	Illness of the testicles
Knap-weed	Catarrh
Lady's help	White's leucorrhea
Lady's mantle	Catarrh of the vagina
Lady's slipper (Cypripedium Calceolus)	Menstrual trouble
Water-plantain (Alisma Plantago)	Labour pains
Five-finger grass, cinquefoil	
(Potentilla Reptans)	Women's disease
Gale	Mouth-odour
Ermander (Teucrium/Chamaedrys)	Gout
Daisy (Bellis Perennis)	Anal pains
Wall-cress (Arabis Hirsuta)	Urinal Passage

The Moor Natures Healing Miracle

Goose rue	*Spermatorrhoea*
Wild wheat	*Gout*
Herb used against the gout	*Gout*
Loosestrife (Lysimachia Vulgaris)	*Scurf, dandruff*
Bell-flowers (Campanula)	*Tendon sheath*
Water hyssop (Gratiola Offinalis)	*Paralyses*
Golden-rod (Solidago)	*Gastric juices*
Gottesknap	*Backache*
Grindeliakraut	*Asthma*
Ground-ivy (Glechoma Hederacea)	*Eyes*
(Afuga)	*Liver*
"Good Henry"	*Gout*
Hawk-week (Hieracium)	*Nose-bleeding*
Oats (Wild)	*Intestinal catarrh*
Crowfoot, stinging	*Liver*
Crowfoot, flabby	*Gall bladder*
Hazelwort (Asarum Europaeum)	*(Emetic)*
Hare-foot	*(Wounds)*
Rest harrow	*Bladder ailment*
(Glecoma/hederacea)	*Whites (Vaginal discharge)*
Bilberry (Vaccinium/Myrtillus)	*Diabetes mellitus*
Health-myrtle	*Dropsy*
Heath-rose (Helianthemum Fumana)	*Remedy for wounds*
Heidnischwundkraut	*Gout*
Scutellaria	*Lung*
Meadow-saffron (Colchicum Autumnale)	*Gastric complaint*
Raspberry bush (Rubus Idaeus)	*Stomach*
Primrose (Primula)	*Cough*
Shepherd's purse (Capsella Bursa Pastoris)	*Asthma*
Hemp-nettle (Galeopsis)	*Tooth ache*
Col'ts foot (Tussilago Farfara)	*Asthma*
Bur-reed	*Nerves*
Staggerwort (Senecio Jacobaea)	*Eyes*
Currant-bush (Ribes)	
"Gichtbeere" - Black currant	*Gout*
John's wort (Hypericum)	*Burns*
Calamus	*Gastric bleeding*
Camomile	*Inflammations*
Mallow (Malva Neglecta)	*Loosens the phlegm*
Cat-thyme (Teucrium Marum)	*Constipation*
Cat's foot (Gnaphalium Dioicum)	*Stomach*
Chervil (Chaerophyllum, Anthriscus, Myrrhis)	*Herpes*

Herbs of the Moor and their Indications

Clover (Trifolium)	Boils, apostemes
Burdock (Arctium)	Swelling
Orchis, broad-leaved	Disease of the testes
Orchis, flesh-coloured	Night sweats
Kopfbinse	Scurf, dandruff
Crakeberry, crowberry (Empetrum)	Urinal passage
Curly-mint (Mentha Crispa)	Stomach
Kreisdorn	Bilious complaint
Cross-flower, milkwort (Polygala Vulgaris)	Abscess, boils
Stunted pine	(Healing baths)
Pond-weeds, general	Nerves
Pond-weed (Potamogeton) with dense foliage	Stomach
Pond-week (Potamogeton), floating	Gullet
Lousewort (Pedicularis)	Skin diseases
Liverleaf (Hepatica Nobilis)	Liver
Water-liverwort	Kidney
Mountain-pine	Lung-catarrh
Flax-weed (Linaria)	Phlegm
"Lily rush"	Gall bladder
lint-(Moor-) Kraut	Rheumatism
Spoonwort (Cochlearia)	Uterine Ligaments
Dandelion (Leontodon Taraxacum)	Intestinal complaint
Lung-flower, marsh gentian (Gentiana Pneumonanthe) hemoptysis	Spitting of blood;
Madessus	Fever
Mallow (Malva)	Herpes, wet
Marguerite (Bellis Perennis)	Herpes, dry
Marzenbecher	Change of life
Masterwort	Fever
Melissa, balm-gentle (Melissa Officinalis)	Heart
Skirret (Sium)	Nose
Mints (Menthae)	Stomach
Mohrenweizen	Cough
(Orchis)	Night sweats
Mohrwurz	Troublesome complaints
due	
	to age
Lofty bulrush	Hoarseness
Morel (Morchella Esculenta)	Testicular illness
Moor-(Lint) Kraut	Rheumatism

The Moor Natures Healing Miracle

"Moor fungi"	Pulmonary disease
"Moor mushrooms"	Cancer of the oesophagus
"Moor rose", "Water lily" (Nymphaea)	Heart-ache, cardialgia
"Moor pepper"	Heat flushes
"Moor-spider-wort"	Eczema
Moorberry, mossberry, cranberry (Vaccinium Oxycoccus)	
"Moss garlic"	Paralyses
Narcissae	Complaints due to age
Adder's wort, bistort	Sciatica
(Polygonum Bistorta)	
Pinks (Dianthus)	Gout
Bennet, avens, (Geum/Urbanum)	Neuritis
Nettles (Urtica)	Gums
"Sneeze-milfoil"	Eczemas
Hellebore (Helleborus)	Prostrate
Agrimony (Latin; agrimonia;	Leanness
(Greek: argemone)	
Peony (Paeonia) (Gout-rose)	Gravel
Catch-fly (Lychnis Viscaria)	Gout
Azure molinia	Barrenness
Red whortleberry or red bilberry,	Bronchitis
cowberry (Vaccinium Vitis Idaea)	
Wild thyme	Urine
Common tansy (Tanacetum Vulgare)	Headache
Crake-berry (Empetrum Nigrum)	Worms
Rue (Ruta Graveolens)	Sore throat
Stork's bill (Erodium Cicutarium)	Bleedings, haemorrhage
Ox-eye	Pain in the chest
Marigold (Calendula)	Wounds
Ritterklee	Liver
Knight's spur	Ovaries
Rohrglanzgras	Cough
Reed-mace (Typha)	Gout
Reed (Phragmites Communis)	Sciatica
Rosemary (Rosmarinus)	Rheumatism
(Wild rosemary)	
Sept-foil, tormentil;	Lumbar weakness
Herb-robert (Geranium Robertianum)	Diarrhoea
Saatwucherblume	Gout
Sage (Salvia)	Bleedings
Sanicle (Sanicula Europaea)	Sore throat
Sorrel (Rumex)	Eczema
	Bowels

- 11 -

Herbs of the Moor and their Indications

Wood sorrel (Oxalis Acetosella)	Tongue
Schachblume	Palate
Shave-(or pewter-)grass (Equisetum)	Tuberculosis
Milfoil (Achillea Millefolium)	Flatulence
Reed (Phragmites, Arundo)	Palsy
Schlammhalm	Consumption
Mud-shave-grass	Tuberculosis
Cowslip (Primula Officinalis)	Cough
White rose celandine (Chelidonium Maius)	Haemorrhoids
Flag, flower de luce (Iris) blue	Diabetes
Yellow water-lily) (Nuphar Luteum)	Cold (in the head) running of the nose, nasal catarrh
(Common) white water-lily (Nymphaea Alba)	Hoarseness
Sedge-grass (Carex)	Skin disease
Sedge, bloated	Eczemas
Sedge, "Davalls"	Herpes
Sedge, yellow	Dandruff
Sedge, high	Scab, mange
Daphne	Paralyses
(Saponaria)	Flatulence
Soapwort	Purification of the blood
Celery (Apium Graveolens)	Hormonal disorders
Chickweed (Trientalis Europaea)	Sweat
Sundew (Drosera), carnivorous	Eyes
Spiraea	Purgative
Spiessmoos	Rheumatism
Rib-grass (Plantago Lanceolata) phlegm	Obstruction caused by
Mocker	Rheumatism
Holly (Iles Aquifolium)	Women's disease
(Silene Armeria)	Jaundice
Marsh-moss (Mnium Unulatum)	Gout
"Stink-morel	Gout
Stork's bill (Geranium)	Barrenness
Grass of parnassus	Facial redness
"Marsh finger-fern"	Women's disease
"Marsh-dragon-wort"	Fever
Marsh-arrow-grass	Influenza
Marsh-marigold (Caltha Palustris)	Bleedings
Marsh-fern (Aspidium Thelypteris)	Wounds

The Moor Natures Healing Miracle

Marsh-sulphurwort

Grass of parnassus
   (Parnassia Palustris) growing in marshes
Sumpfkopf
"Marsh-horse-thistle"
"Marsh galium"
Red rattle
"Marsh-chickweed"
Marsh-(or wild) rosemary
   (Ledum Palustre)
"Marsh rosemary tad-pipe
   (Equisetum Limosum)
"Marsh milfoil"
"Marsh-sedge-grass"
"Marsh-violet"
"Marsh-forget-me-not"
"Marsh-willow-herb"
Mudwort
Marsh-woundwort, clown's all-heal
   (Stachys Palustris)
Glyceria
Dead-nettle (Lamium)
Water milfoil (Myriophyllum)
Centaury (Erythraea)
Bulrush
   Thyme (Thymus Vulgaris)
Peat-moss (Sphagnum Cymbifolium)

Wood-scabious
rash"

Common club-moss; wolf's claw
"Peat-grass"
"Peat-lily"
Tormentil
"Water's edge veronica"
rhoids
Violet (Moor-violet)
Forget-me-not (Myosotis)

Knot-grass (Polygonum Avicularia)
Juniper (Iuniperus)

Neuralgic pains in the joints;
(Articular rheumatism)

Facial redness
Arthrosis
Sore feet
Stomach
Skin-disease
Fatigue

Nerves

Lung
Stomach
Small-pox
Eruption; rash
eyes
Cramp
Nettle-rash (urticaria)

Dropsy
Diet
Urethra
Fever
Constipation

Liver
Change of colour
concerning the skin
German measles; "rose

roseola
Sore feet
Night sweats
Bleedings
Dysentery
(Bleeding) piles; haemor-

Bleeding of the nose
Pains in the joints;
arthralgia
Glands
Circulatory disorders

Herbs of the Moor and their Indications

Sweet william	Complaints due to old age
Water-violet (Hottonia Palustris)	Cough
Water-fennel	Stomach
Water-lily	Hoarseness
Duck-weed (Lemna)	Hoarseness
Water-mint (Mentha Aquatica)	Intestine
Water-weed, anacharis (Elodea Canadensis)	Facial redness
Water-pepper, smartweed (Polygonum Hydropiper)	Urine
Water-hemlock (Utricularia)	Dandruff
Water-starwort (Callitriche Vernalis)	Pustules
Willow (Salix)	Rheumatism
Willow-weed (Lythrum)	Rheumatism
Great burnet (Sanguisorba Officinalis)	Wounds
Water-horehound	Women's disease
Wolf's bane	Health troubles due to accidents
Cotton-grass, broad-leaved	Belly
Cotton-grass, vaginated	Anus
Anthyllis	Wounds
Tansy	Colics
Bryony (Bryonia)	Gout
Chicory	Kidney catarrh
Common horse-tail	Stomach
Twayblade (Listera Ovata)	Intestine
Bur marigold (Bidens Cernua)	Dysentery
Bur marigold, three-cleft	Circulatory disorders
And many others	

As the foregoing herbs and plants including many others, sank into the Moor thousands of years ago and due to the natural preservation of their many healing substances in a live and active state, a profound healing effect on the whole body results.

Unlike the single application of a herbal healing substance which can in many instances cause a loss of the natural equilibrium within the organism, the Moor treatments embrace the whole range of various healing agents derived from the many hundreds of Moor herbs and plants in their natural wholeness and totality.

According to scientific opinions the therapeutic action of the Moor is for the most part considered a quintuple (Fivefold) one namely; astringent, absorbent, ion-exchanging, hormonal and inflammation restraining.

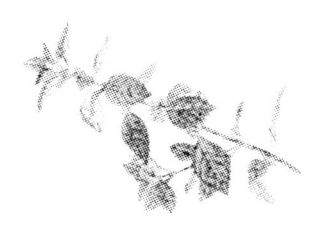

I quote from Professor F. Zaribricky, M.D., D.V.M. former President of the International Society for Research on Moor; "Practical experience has taught for a long time that a certain kind of moor as a God-created natural healing agent is, in its totality, effective against an astonishing number of diseases".

Neydharting Healing Moor has proven highly successful in the treatment of the following complaints:

Acne
Arthritis
Arthrosis
Athlete's foot
Bladder infections
Burns
Circulatory disturbances
Climacteric complaints

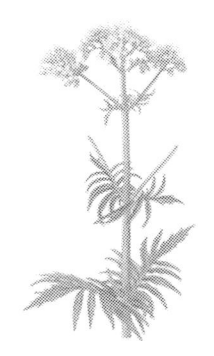

Colic
Colitis
Degenerative ailments
Duodenitis, duodenal ulcers
Endometritis
Enteritis
Enterocolitis
Follow-up treatment of polio victims
Gall-bladder complaints
Gastric-hyper-acidity
Gastritis
Gout
Gynaecological complaints, chronic
Infertility
Inflamed joints
Inflammations of gastric mucosa, peptic ulcers
Inflammations of the genital tract
Inflammations of the intervertebral discs
Inflammations pelvic tissue
Inflammation of the renal pelvis
Kidney disorders
Liver complaints
Lumbago
Menopausal complaints
Menstrual disorders
Metabolic disturbances
Muscular strain
Myalgia
Neuralgia
Neuritis
Ovarian disorders
Phlebitis
Piles
Prostatitis
Psoriasis

Rheumatism
Rheumatoid arthritis
Rheumatoid myositis
Scar retraction
Sciatica
Severe constipation
Skin diseases, various
Spondylarthritis
Sterility
Stiff joints
Treatment of the consequences of accidents
Uterine disorders
Vaginal catarrh
Vaginitis

Indications for Moor Therapy

Indications

Acne vulg
Adhesions
Adipositas (fatness)
Amenorrhoea (Absence or abnormal stoppage of the menses)
Amoebiasis
Arthritis chronic
Arthritis
Arthrosis
Blepharitis (inflammation of the eyelids)
Purification of the blood
Bursitis
packs
Caries
mouthwash
Cervicitis (inflammation of the cervix uteri)

Therapy

Moor mask for the face
Moor baths (packs)
Moor packs; baths

Moor baths; drink
Moor drinking cure
Moor baths; Moor packs
Moor baths; Moor packs
Moor bath (hot and warm)

Moor eye drops
Moor drinking cure
Moor partial baths and

Rinsing with Moor

"Vaginal douche";Moor baths

Cholecystitis (inflammation of the gall bladder)	Moor drinking cure; Moor Packs
Coccygodynia (pain in the coccyx)	Moor baths
Colitis	Moor drinking cure
Comedones mask	Moor face wash; Moor for the face
Conjunctivitis	Moor eye drops
Contusion (bruise)	Moor partial baths; packs
Dysmenorrhoea (painful menstruation)	Moor baths; packs; drink
Endometritis (inflammation of the membrane of the uterus)	Moor drinking cure; Moor baths
Enteritis (inflammation of the intestine)	Moor drinking cure
Gastritis	Moor drinking cure
Gingivitis (inflammation of the gum)	Moor gingival paste
Haemorrhoids	Moor sitzbaths (cool)
Hyperacidity	Moor drinking cure (after eating)
Hypermenorrhoea (abnormally profuse or persistent menstruation)	Moor baths (cool); drink
Intercostal-neuralgia	Moor baths
Climacteric troubles	Moor sitzbaths; full baths (luke warm); drinking cure
Lumbago (backache)	Moor pack (hot)
Meteorism (abnormal presence of gas in the gastro-intestinal tract)	Moor drinking cure
Metritis (inflammation of the uterus)	Moor baths; drink
Metrorrhagia (an abnormal uterine haemorrhage)	Moor baths; drink
Myalgia (muscle pain)	Moor baths (lukewarm)
Nephropathy (disease of the kidneys)	Moor partial baths; drink
Neuralgia	Moor baths
Neuritis (inflammation of the nerve)	Moor baths
Constipation	Moor drinking cure

Phlebitis (inflammation of a vein)	*Moor partial baths; drink*
Polyarthritis (inflammation of numerous joints) drink	*Moor baths; Moor packs;*
Polyneuritis (inflammation of numerous nerves) drink	*Moor baths; Moor packs;*
Prostatitis	*Intestinal Moor baths; Moor sitz baths; drinking cure*
Psoriasis (a skin disease characterised by scaly red patch formations on the extensor surfaces of the body)	*Moor baths; drinking cure*
Spasms	*Moor baths*
Sterility	*Moor baths; packs; Moor drinking cure*
Stomach-ulcers	*Moor drinking cure*
Vulvitis (inflammation of the vulva)	*Moor sitzbaths; douche*
Vulvovaginitis (inflammation of the vulva and vagina)	*Moor sitzbaths; douche*

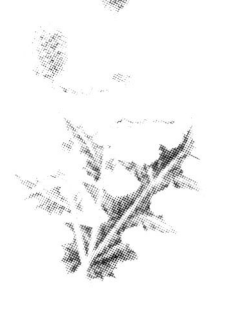

"The Creator in his infinite goodness has made remedies for men and animals in the most insignificant looking things, at which modern man indifferently goes by and which he even despises and looks down upon"

(Pastor Sebastian Kneipp, Priest Physician)

Quinta Essentia

Since time immemorial mankind has searched for plant medicines to heal in times of sickness and injury. Herbs are man's oldest system of healing; ancient records list herbs and plants for medicinal purposes, information was also in cluded as to how to identify and use them.

Only plants and herbs can absorb inorganic materials and convert them into organic matter; plants and herbs change dead and decayed matter into living substances, this ongoing process is virtually impossible for man to duplicate. Every second of every day plants and herbs through almost infinitesimal root hairs discharge chemical acids which have the power of breaking down essential mineral substances which the plant absorbs.

From earliest times man has found his food and medicine in the plant kingdom. Today science has begun research into natural substances in an effort to find safer medicinal alternatives to synthetic materials. As a result of this research more is coming to light as to how plants and herbs of traditional folk medicine worked.

The scientists at the Neydharting Moor have dedicated themselves in producing and developing a superior range of natural Moor treatments which over many years of use have proven their healing efficacy. Over one thousand different plant and herbal species can be found on the Moor and due to natural preservation of the whole plants, i.e., roots, blooms, stalks, fruits, leaves, tubers and seeds in the process of decomposition, the mud and waters contain a wealth of vitamins, minerals, trace and micro-elements, hormone, enzyme and antibiotic agents.

After careful observation of my patients who have been taking especially the Moor herbal drink and Baths as recommended by Professor Stober over a regular period of time, besides the many healing and curative benefits, the Moor is capable of protecting the body against stress in a natural way.

It is my belief that certain agents in the Moor act as adaptogens whose purpose is to supply energy to the cells permitting them to function more efficiently when under adverse stressful conditions. Furthermore, the Moor Drink and Bath works indirectly via complex regulatory systems of the body which involve the whole organism, this being the reason why the Moor is so effective in such a wide range of health problems. The Moor therefore, assists the body to correct and balance itself through stimulating the energy supply to every cell which in turn allows the body's natural and inherent capacity of self-regeneration to function.

A certain vital force or subtle healing energy is undoubtedly present in the Moor, many of the miracle cures that have taken place could be put down to this.

Considering in every way, the Moor is the result of a natural process of events which have been taking place over millions of years and as nothing is added or taken away the Moor can certainly be looked upon as totally holistic in every meaning of the word.

"In the quintessence of the black moor nature brings to us a gift from god. The strength of this quintessence of the black moor remains unbroken only in the naturally pure state".

(Professor Otto Stober, Pioneer of Moor Research)

Healing Herbs from the Moor

When first visiting the Neydharting Moor one is attracted by the deep, rich and velvety blackness of the mud and waters resulting from natural continuous organic changes over thousands of years of the multitudinous numbers of plants and fauna which have sunk into the waters.

In view of the vast number of medicinal herbs whose wealth of therapeutic properties the mud and waters hold, it can quite easily be perceived why such healing miracles occur time and time again.

A Partial Contents List of the Neydharting Moor

Devil's bit	*Oak-wort*	*Aconite*
Pearl wort	*Iron wort*	*Gentian*
Elecampane	*Strawberry Plant*	*Fumitory*
Horehound	*Alderbush*	*Ferns, bracken*
Wood angelica	*Black alder*	*Dyer's weed*
Stonewort	*Fennel*	*Butterwort*
Arnica	*Bogbean marsh trefoil*	*Soft rush*
Dwarf elder root	*Fletchbinse*	*Fly-orchis*
Eyebright	*Knap-weed*	*Ladys help*
Brooklime	*Ladys mantle*	*Ladys slipper*
Bennet, avens	*Water plantain*	*Fuve-finger grass*
Badekraut	*Gale*	*Germander*
Valerian	*Daisy*	*Wall-cress*
Bear's Bilberry	*Goose rue*	*Wild wheat*
Club Moss	*Loosestrife*	*Broom*
Barlauch	*Various-leaved canary grass*	*Bell-flowers*
Sweet basil	*Water hyssop*	*Golden-rod*
Mugwort	*Gottesknab*	*Grindeliakraut*
Bog-asphodel	*Ground-ivy*	*Aiuga*

Consound	"Good Henry"	Hawk-weed
Common Broom	Oats (wild)	Crow-foot(stinging)
Burnet saxifrage	Hazelwort	Crow foot (flabby)
Henbane	Hare-foot	Rest harrow
Moss rush	Glecoma	Heather
Bindengewachse	Bilberry	Heath-myrtle
Birches	Heindnischwundkraut	Heath rose
Buck-bean	Scutellaria	Meadow saffron
Cuckoo-flower	Raspberry Bush	Primrose
Flowering Bush	Shepherd's purse	Hemp-nettle
Finger fern	Colt's foot	Bur-reed
Blood wort	Staggerwort	Curranbush
Purple loosestrife	John's wort	Calamus
Fenugreek	Camomile	Mallow
Brown wort	Cat-thyme	Cat's foot
Brennkraut	Chervil	Clover
Bramble	Burdock	Kopfbinse
Bruesch	Orchis (brown Leaved)	Crowberry
Water-cress	Orchis (flesh coloured)	Cross-flower
Stunted-pine	Butter flower marigold	Pond weed(general)
Marsh mallow root	Pond weed (dense foliage)	Pond weed(floating)
Lousewort	Liverleaf	Water liverwort
Mountain-pine	Flax-weed	"Lily-rush"
Lint kraut	Spoonwort	Dandelion
Lung flower	Lung wort	Madesuss
Marguerite	Marzenbecher	Golden saxifrage
Mints	Mohrenweizen	Orchis
Mohwurz	Lofty bulrush	Morel
Moor lintkraut	Moor fungi	Moor mushrooms
Moor rose	Moor pepper	Cotton-grass
Moor spiderwort	Moorberry cranberry	Moss-garlic
Narcissae	Adder's wort	Pinks
Bennet, avens	Nettles	Sneeze-milfoil
Hellebore	Agrimony	Red bilberry
Couch grass	Wild thyme	Common tansy
Crake-berry	Rue	Stork's bill
Sedge reed grass	Rikoraris	Ox-eye
Marigold	Ritterklee	Knight's spur
Rohrglanzgras	Reed-mace	Reeds (various)
Rosemary	Sept-foil	Herb-Robert
Saatwucherblume	Sage	Wood-sorrel
Schachblume	Shave grass	Milfoil
Hemlock	Schlammhalm	Mud-shave grass

Hemlock	Schlammhalm	Mud-shave grass
Cowslip	White rose	Celandine
Iris	Sword flag	Yellow water lily
White water lily	Sedge-grass	Sedge, bloated
Sedge "Davalls"	Sedge yellow	Sedge high
Daphne	Saponaria	Soapwort
Celery	Chickweed	Sundew
Spriraea	Spiessmoos	Rib-grass
"Mocker"	Holly	Silene armeria
Starwort	Marsh moss	"Stink-morel"
Stork's bill	Grass of parnassus	Marsh finger fern
Marsh dragon wort	Marsh arrow grass	Marsh fern
Marsh sulphurwort	Marsh marigold	Sumpfkopf
Marsh horse thistle	Marsh galium	Red rattle
Marsh chickweed	Marsh rosemary(wild)	Marsh reed grass
Marsh rosemary	Tad-pipe	Marsh milfoil
Marsh sedge grass	Marsh violet	Marsh forget-me-not
Marsh willow herb	Mudwort	Marsh-woundwort
Glyceria	Dead-nettle	Water milfoil
Centaury	Bulrush	Thyme
Peat-moss	Wood scabious	Common club moss
Peat grass	Peat lily	Tormentil
Water's edge veronica	Moor-violet	Forget-me-not
Knot grass	Juniper	Woodruff
Sweet william	Water violet	Water fennel
Water lily	Duck weed	Water mint
Anarcharis	Water pepper	Water hemlock
Bladder wort	Water starwort	Willow
Willow-weed	Great burnet	Water-horehound
Wolf's bane	Cotton-grass (broad leaved)	Tansy
Anthyllis	Cotton-grass (vaginated)	Bryony
Chicory	Common horse tail	Twayblade
Bur marigold (various)	Wild asparagus	Pimpernel
Genista	Delphinium	Water parsnip
Radish	Sundew	Water moss
Curly-mint	Kreisdorn	Sand-reed
Sanicle	Sorrel	

The Moor Research Scientists in conjunction with the Austrian Government are conducting on-going analysis of the Moor and have estimated there to be at least another 400 species of FLORA in the Moor of Neydharting.

Organic Substances

Organic sulphur
Bitumen
Resins
Pectins
Hums substances
Fulvo acids
Lingnine

R..G. acids
Starch
Balm
Salicylate
Xylose
Cellulose & many more

Nitrogen compounds
Various types of wax
Fats
Amino acids
Oxalic acids
Humic acids
Fatty acids (both saturated & unsaturated)
Sugar
Volatile oils
Biopterin
Tannic acid
Etheric oil

Trace Elements

Boron
Zirconium
Silver
Copper
Iodine
Cobalt

Strontium
Chromium
Gold
Manganese
Iron
Brass & many more

Biologically Active Matter

Natural antibiotics
Estrones
Various Pro and Active vitamins

Taking the Healing Waters

The Moor Bath

Many thousands of people have experienced the curative effects of the Moor Bath and Drink. At one time it was necessary to travel to Austria for treatment; fortunately, the treatments are now available here in the UK for people to take in their own homes.

In one year alone some 7,000,000 Moor Baths were dispensed in Austria which proves the immense healing efficacy and popularity that the Neydharting Moor enjoys.

The Moor Bath in liquid suspension was developed by Professor Stober. The skin is able to absorb through its pores the various dissolved healing substances which are taken into the body to carry out their curative action.

Amongst the many therapeutic agents which the bather absorbs are bitumens, hormones, micro-trace elements and humic acids which produces an exchange reaction of ions. Certain fatty acids and fat soluble substances allow for greater and easier absorption through the skin. The Moor Bath when dissolved in water contains many healing factors which are quickly absorbed by the blood vessels into the system to carry out their precious healing work.

The therapeutic indications for the Moor Bath are arthritis, rheumatic complaints, inflamed muscles and joints, traumatic effects of injuries and accidents, gynaecological, hormonal, menopausal and other female problems, prostate inflammation, skin troubles, obesity and metabolic disorders, immune deficiency illness, insomnia, circulatory complaints especially poor circulation, varicose veins etc.

The therapeutic efficacy of the Moor Bath consists of a thermal, mechanical and chemical action, the chemical effects being of considerable importance especially in the treatment of arthritic, rheumatic and gynaecological problems.

The question "Why are the substances dissolved in the Moor therapeutically effective?" is largely unanswered, however Professor Dr J Kowarschik of the International Moor Research Institute, cites two main areas of interest:

Nerve Stimulant

The substances cling to the skin or penetrate partially between the epidermis cells of the skin. A binding process with albumin in the skins follows. Of greater importance, however are the effects it seems to have on the vegetative nervous system. The fibres of this system, situated between the cells of the epidermis, are stimulated directly. Eventually all organs in contact with this system are influenced neurally.

Hormonal Effects

As the Moors healing substances penetrate into the capillaries, they are taken up by the bloodstream, and released into the circulation. As to which of the Moor's substances penetrate into the circulation, this can only be established by further research.

One doctor has shown that in the use of Neydharting Moor Baths the amount of cortisones produced are sufficient to achieve a complete cortisone effect in the treatment of joint disorders. Another specialist has proved that during the course of Neydharting Moor treatments, oestrogen hormones are increased as is the excretion of progesterone, which stimulates the activities of the ovaries.

A Moor Bath is easily prepared by adding the required liquid to the bath water which has a temperature of not more than 36 - 37 celsius. It is most important that the Moor Liquid is thoroughly dispersed in the water so as to enable the healing substances complete absorption into the skin.

The duration of the bath should last no longer than fifteen to twenty minutes, after which the bather should neither towel dry or shower, merely covering the body with a large towel or bathrobe and retiring to bed for approximately one hour or better still, the bath can be taken last thing at night; the reason being that during rest the various healing agents that are still in contact with the skin continue their action of penetration thus maintaining their healing work on the organism. It is possible for the Moor's healing effects to continue for up to twenty four hours following the bath.

In treating chronic conditions it is recommended that twenty one baths are taken either on a daily basis or every other day. It is often necessary to repeat this regime several times over a period of many months in order to obtain good results, furthermore, once a course has been commenced it should not be interrupted.

A healing reaction to the Moor Bath is often experienced. This should not be taken as a bad sign, to the contrary, any healing reaction or crisis is a sign that nature is attempting a cure. The direction of cure is always from above down, from within out and from an important organ to a lesser important organ, also the symptoms should clear in the reverse order in which they presented themselves.

The various healing reactions can manifest in increased aches and pains and exacerbation of existing symptoms. Also parts of the body which were previously symptomless become uncomfortable and painful, these healing reactions may quite quickly clear only to reappear later on into the treatment. However, whatever form the healing crisis takes it is constructive and necessary if nature is allowed, and given time to heal the diseased organism.

The Moor Bathing liquid can also be used for sitz (hip), hand and foot baths. Also, it is ideal for compresses to apply in specific areas of the body such as shoulders, back, arms, knees and legs. In this case the Moor liquid is heated in a suitable container or saucepan to a temperature of 40°celsius, a cloth which has previously been wrung out in hot water is then covered with the heated Moor liquid which should resemble a paste. It is then applied directly to the affected area and covered with a warm blanket or better still, a heating pad so as to retain the thermal effects as long as possible. The compress should remain on the respective part of the body for approximately thirty minutes. It is most important that the Moor compress should not become too hot.

People with high blood pressure should take great care when undergoing the Moor Bathing treatment. If in doubt, it is advisable to consult their physician, however, observations by Neydharting Spa physicians showed that normal blood pressure could be achieved in those whose blood pressure was high through taking the Moor Bath provided that the water for this purpose is pleasantly warm and not hot.

Skin Brushing

So as to improve the absorption of the Moor Bath through the skin I recommend a dry skin brushing of the whole body prior to bathing. Dry brushing is a form of self massage which is most stimulating. It eliminates the build up of dead cells which the skin is constantly shedding. Dry brushing improves the blood and lymph circulation and should of course for this reason alone be practised daily even when not taking the Moor Bath. However, if taking the full twenty one day Moor Bathing cure on every other night, do not skin brush the morning following the Moor Bath otherwise you will disturb the fine particles left on your skin from the Bath and in doing so lose some of the benefits of the Moor Bath.

You will require a pure natural-bristle body brush, the long handle type preferably, with a detachable handle.

It is most important to keep your brush clean as it is loosening and lifting off dead skin cells and other impurities. **NB**, The Moor Bathing liquid does not stain clothing, towels or baths.

The dry brushing technique is as follows:

Remove the long handle. Commence by brushing your feet, working along the soles, toes, tops of feet and ankles. Use a firm stroking movement: after having treated the feet and ankles, brush upwards from ankles to thighs; next brush your hands, fingers and palms, sweeping up the arms from wrists to elbows and upwards to shoulders. Next brush across the tops of your shoulders, covering the back of the neck and front and sides downwards towards the upper chest.

Next treat the front of your body: brush lightly across your chest; avoiding the breasts, moving down to the abdomen brushing in ever increasing circles commencing at the naval in a clockwise direction continue all around the abdomen in this manner, after which commencing at the right side of your waist, brush in small circles round the top to your hip and over the buttock : repeat these movements to the opposite side. Lastly, to brush the back you will require the long handle replaced in your brush, working from the top of your back backwards and forwards, and downwards to your buttocks. Change your hands frequently when covering the back. This whole procedure should only take 5-6 minutes, even less once you become accustomed to the various movements, your skin and body is now in a receptive state to absorb the many healing and nourishing substances of the Moor Bath.

"Let Mother Nature show you the true path to health"
"Dr Benedict Lust"

Moor Foot Bath

It has been recognised for thousands of years by many civilisations that there is a relationship between areas on the feet and the body's organs, nerves and limbs. In many countries doctors have integrated holistic therapies into their medicinal clinics, the practice of reflexology being one such valid therapy.

The Moor Foot Bath is an excellent way of stimulating the reflex points on the feet; taken before retiring it can alleviate sleep disorders, poor circulation, disorders of the stomach and intestines, kidneys and bladder etc.

The Bath can also strengthen weak muscles in the feet. Healing substances in the Moor are absorbed through the soles into the blood vessels and nerves which reach the whole organism.

For a Moor Foot Bath: fill a suitable kitchen bowl with warm water and add approximately a quarter of a cup of the Moor Bath Liquid making sure it is thoroughly dissolved. Allow the feet to remain in the Bath for 10-15 minutes after which pat dry and massage well into the soles and upper area of the feet and ankles the Moor Life Body Cream or Moor Massage Oil. By treating feet the Moor way the entire body benefits.

Moor Arm Bath

This bath favourable influences the heart, improves the circulation and relieves cramps and inflammations of the fingers lymph vessels and joints. Prepare in exactly the same manner as the Foot Bath. The water however, for this purpose, should be cool. Bending the elbows, place both arms into the water allowing it to reach just below the shoulders. The arms should remain in the water for 5-10 minutes after which pat dry and with long sweeping strokes massage the Moor Life Oil into each arm commencing at the fingers and finishing below the shoulders.

Hip or Sitz Bathing

A baby's bath is excellent for this purpose. Should one not be available an ordinary bath will suffice, however, the knees must be up and flexed thus allowing only the buttocks and feet in contact with the water which should reach the level of the hips or pelvic bones. It is important that the water temperature does not exceed 30 celsius. Use approximately a quarter of a cup of the Moor Bathing Liquid ensuring thorough dispersal of the liquid in the water. Sitting in the water with thighs flexed and open splash with the hands the lower pelvic regions; after approximately 10 minutes wrap a large bath towel round the waist and rest for one hour.

This method of bathing has a profound healing, strengthening and rejuvenating effect on all the organs situated within the pelvis and is indicated for the following disorders; haemorrhoids; pruritus; cystitis; prostatitis; bladder weakness; kidney problems; sexual troubles including impotency and frigidity, female diseases such as vaginitis, leucorrhoea, thrush and menopausal problems etc. In conjunction with the Moor Bouquet many disturbing and tenacious diseases of the pelvic organs can be eradicated.

The Moor Drink

The Moor Herbal Drink known as the Moor Bouquet is hygienically processed from specific areas of the Moor, diluted with Moor water and finally pasteurised. It contains a wealth of active healing substances which are easily absorbed through the gastro intestinal tract and taken thereby to every part of the organism.

The therapeutic efficacy of the Moor Bouquet is a result of the following bio-available processes:

The volatile oils, lipoids, waxes and resins contained in Nedharting Healing Moor gently cover the mucous membranes of the stomach and the sensitive inner walls of the intestines with a fine protective film.

The healing power of the Moor therefore actively neutralizes and combats inflammatory processes in the stomach and intestines. As a result of the Moor's energetic surface activity, poisons and gasses are absorbed and rendered harmless.

Neydharting Healing Moor is an excellent antacid, thus excess stomach acidity is absorbed. This normalises the patient's gastric juices and secretions.

The Moor also effectively encourages the self-regulation of intestinal flora, whose proper functioning is an absolutely essential part of good health.

Moreover, the Bouquet and Herbal Drink provides the body with valuable restorative and revitalising substances.

Scientists at the Austrian Moor Research Institute have been able to identify a wealth of bio-chemical agents in the Moor Bouquet. There are of course many other healing substances which in time no doubt, will be identified.

General Analysis of the Moor Ingredients

Alkali salts, aluminium hydrates, formic acid, amino acids, ammonium, inorganic sulphur, antibiotics, malic acids, arabinose, volatile oils, balsam, succinic acid, biopterin, bitumen, bitter principles, butyric acid, chlorides, chlorates, iron oxides, albumin, acetic acid, colouring matters, ferro (iron II) and ferri (iron III) salts, fats, fat acids (for instances, vitamin groups F), folic acids, fructoses, fulvo acids, galactan, tannic acids, glucosides, glutamic acids, resins, hemicelluloses, hexosans, hormones, humins, humic acids, humolignin, humus accompanying substances, hyper sulphides, inosites, iodine salts, potassium oxide, calcium oxide, carotenes, silicic acid, carbonic acid, levulinic acids, lignin, magnesium salts, manganese compounds, mannan, metasilicic acid, methane, lactic acid, monosaccharides, sodium compounds, oils, organic sulphates, organic sulphides, oxalic acid, pantothenic acid, pectins, penicillia, pentosans, phosphoric acids, protein, propionic acid, purine bodies, rhamnose, hormone-substances, saponins, salicylates, hydrogen sulphide, silicon compounds, starch, nitrogen compounds, trace elements, boron, barium, chromium, copper, titanium, vanadium, zirconium, strontium, uric acids, vitamins, waxes, xylose, cellulose, various kinds of sugar, and others.

Professor Stober states in his book 'Die Moorfibel' that the Moor Bouquet contains the active substances of some three hundred healing plants, little wonder that the Moor Drink benefits such a wide diversity of health problems.

Perhaps the most spectacular healing effects resulting from taking the Moor Bouquet are those conditions affecting the gastro intestinal tract especially duodenal ulcers, gastritis, stomach acidity, colitis, irritable bowel syndrome and various other digestive and bowel disorders. Dr I. Kallus, Senior Medical Officer at the General Hospital, Klagenfurt, Austria, has cited 4,000 cases of gastro-duodenal ulcers which he treated with the Moor Bouquet, of those cases, 3,720 were so successful that surgery was considered unnecessary.

It is my conjecture that as well as the many therapeutic effects of the Moor Bouquet, it also acts as a natural chelating medium mainly due to various pectin substances, certain minerals and trace minerals which have the ability to bind and take up unwanted heave toxic metals such as mercury, lead, aluminium and cadmium from the tissues and eliminating them safely from the body.

Heavy toxic metals which unfortunately we are all exposed to are potent and most damaging to the entire functioning of the brain and body. Many scientists believe that heavy toxic metals are responsible for some forms of cancer, cardio-vascular, arterial diseases, also certain neurological illnesses, such as alzheimers disease.

Dr Bircher-Benner, the famous nature cure doctor from Switzerland prescribed the Moor Bouquet to his many patients suffering from various inflammatory conditions of the internal organs resulting in general improvement of symptoms, in some cases within a matter of days.

Over recent years it is a sad medicinal fact that due to the widespread use of antibiotics and sulphonamides the friendly and normal intestinal flora that are so necessary to maintain health are damaged and destroyed. When friendly flora are destroyed by antibiotics there often follows an infection by a virulent (disease producing) bacterial or fungal organism. This organism may have been present in small numbers but held in check by the normal flora. There is ample evidence that much of the beneficial bacteria indigenous to the organism produce and secrete antibiotic like substances. Furthermore, the normal flora through its waste products establishes a medium that is too acid which is not conducive for the growth and development of harmful bacteria. The maintenance of normal flora is an important aspect of the organisms defence, the killing off of normal flora of any region of the body is dangerous and may precipitate serious disease.

Normal and friendly flora equally applies to other parts and areas of the body besides the gastro-intestinal tract, for example, the skin, ears, mouth, urinary system and vagina, all to various degrees rely on friendly flora being present.

The Moor contains many strains of beneficial bacteria and friendly flora, scientists have identified coliform bacteria in the Moor which plays a significant role in the human organism, namely, for the restoration of imbalanced intestinal flora. Dr Wolfgang Paul states in his book 'Healing Earth Moor'.

Observations by Neydharting Moor physicians on patients taking the Moor Bouquet proved that thousands of cases suffering from inflammatory conditions of the joints, muscles, nerves, gastro-intestinal tract, liver, gall-bladder, kidneys, pancreas, prostate, bladder and female reproductive organs, also the mammary glands and tissues were either eliminated or considerably improved.

Furthermore, the Moor Bouquet by virtue of many nutritive substances, hormones, volatile oils, enzymes and other healing factors supply to the blood stream exactly what it requires so as to favourably influence many diseases that afflict the body, even stones in the gall bladder and kidneys can be dissolved given time, this being due to the action of various volatile oils and pectins. Pectins appear to lower blood cholesterol and eliminate bile acids from the intestines which in many cases are the cause of stones in the gall-bladder.

For those who's blood cholesterol is high it would be prudent to take a course of the Moor Bouquet until satisfactory results are obtained after which a reduced dose as a prophylactic measure.

Considering that the Moor Bouquet contains natural hormones, so important where imbalances of the endocrine glands exist, it can be appreciated that many disturbing manifestations which occur during the menopause resulting from hormonal changes can be helped by the Moor Bouquet and Bath

The Moor Bouquet is practically tasteless. It is produced under stringent hygienic conditions under the direction of the Austrian Moor Research Institute including the supervision of the Austrian State. The Bouquet is normally taken three times daily, half-an-hour before meals, one teaspoon can be added to warm water or even tea. A full course can take up to 6 to 8 weeks.

I recommend at all times that the Bouquet is sipped slowly and held in the mouth for a few seconds before swallowing, taken in this manner it will combine with numerous bio-salivary agents thus aiding absorption as well as exerting a beneficial effect on the mouth mucosa in general.

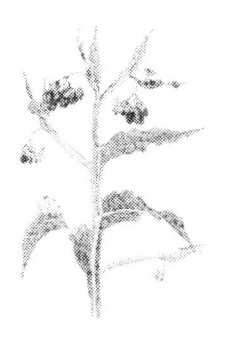

So much of Nature as he is ignorant of, so much of his own mind does he not yet possess and in fine, the ancient precept, "Know Thyself", and the modern precept, "Study Nature" become as last one Maxim ....")

"Ralph Waldo Emerson"

The Moor for Natural Beauty

Some 38 years ago under the direction of Professor Stober the laboratories at the Moor developed a range of natural skin care and beauty products which to this day have remained unchanged.

Besides consisting of all the beneficial healing and organic substances of the Moor, these products have a similar pH factor to that of skin.

They do not contain any harmful chemical matter; every product is hand made and no animal has suffered during the process.

The Moor Life Skin Care products are healthful and beautifying, they slow down ageing of the tissues and rejuvenate the skin. All skin types and all ages, even males can enjoy the pleasure and benefits that the skin care products produce.

The healthy substances of well over 700 herbs and plants in their wholeness and entirety penetrate the skin cells through a unique molecular action which replenishes lost vitality and elasticity to the tissues. The Moor beauty range can certainly be called *"The Living Gift of Nature"* which modern science is unable to come close to.

Emerson wrote: *"Beauty is the pilot of the young soul"*. Beauty is you whatever the age; it is you at your best and most beautiful. There are thousands of types of beauty some of which come from chemists potions and man produced chemicals containing animal parts. I would question however, what damage in the long term can they often produce including premature ageing of the skin.

The beautiful women of bygone days used only lotions and creams made from simple flowers from hedgerow, meadows and streams, yet their natural beauty lingers like the fragrance of immortal perfume. Natural beauty is a gift to be enjoyed through the time honoured Moor Life Natural Beauty range.

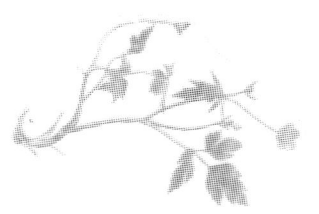

How the Moor Life Skin Care Programme works for everybody and every skin

The four skin care products, used together, constitute a TOTAL SKIN CARE ROUTINE. For best results use only these four products to retain the skin's natural acid mantle.

Neydharting Moor Life Soap/Cleansing Bar

Completely free from alkali (the soap contains only Moor Extract and Cocoa Butter) which means the skin's natural acid mantle is not damaged by washing with this soap. Suitable for normal cosmetic use, sensitive and damaged skin. The Moor soap cares for skin, keeping it smooth and soft and improves circulation, gentle enough even for babie's delicate skin. Ideal for removing make-up.

Neydharting Moor Life Face Mask

This Face Mask is entirely different from any others. It is many thousands of years old and consists only of flowers, plants, grasses and herbs that grow in the unique Neydharting Valley in Austria. The Neydharting Moor Life Face Mask is entirely natural, no chemicals or additive mar the simple essence of the world famous Healing Moor of Neydharting. Many chemicals tests have proved that essential oils, fats, and lipoids are present in the Moor. They occur naturally and do not have to be introduced artificially as in other cosmetics. Being fat soluble, these fatty acids penetrate easily into the skin and for example on the subcutaneous connective tissues, they are extremely valuable for cosmetic purposes. The cream in this tube is dark brown and silky smooth. It is neither perfumed nor glamorous, but the therapeutic properties of the hundreds of different wild flowers gently help to smooth away wrinkles and rejuvenate tired skin in an entirely natural way.

Neydharting Moor Life Face Cream

A very special cream which more than any other Moor preparation illustrates the magic of Nature's own Moor at work, because HERE IS ONE CREAM TO SUIT ALL SKIN TYPES, normal, dry, oily, sensitive and problem skins all respond to Nature's Moor which helps to restore a natural pH balance to achieve a healthy glowing YOU. An ideal moisturiser, make-up base, night cream, throat cream and a safe and effective eye cream too.

The instructions for use of the skin care routine are simple:

1. Clean the skin of the face and neck. (Using Moor Soap).

2. Squeeze just a little of the Face Mask into an egg cup; add 1 teaspoon of water and mix until it just 'hangs' on the fingers or brush.

3. Apply the Face Mask. Leave on for 2-3 minutes for dry skin, or 5-6 minutes for problem skin.

4. Then simply wash off the Face Mask with warm water, and apply the Neydharting Moor Cleansing/Toning Lotion.

5. Finally, smooth on Neydharting Moor Face Cream or Moor Body Cream and gently massage in to the skin.

This treatment improves the blood circulation, braces the skin and gives a feeling of renewed vitality to the face. For a normal undamaged skin, apply the Neydharting Moor Face Mask at 7-10 day intervals. If the skin suffers from acne or other surface blemishes, use daily for 3 weeks then every 3-7 days.

Neydharting Moor Life Body Cream
Naturally antiseptic; apply sparingly. This Body Cream is a highly effective general purpose treatment for the relief of muscular aches and pains, for healing cuts, abrasions, burns, bites, stings and sunburn. Invaluable for acne scars, stretch marks, eczema and nappy rash in babies. It can restore the natural pH balance of the skin. It contains the natural Healing Moor of Neydharting and is pure and a gentle salve for all skin types. It is readily absorbed and non-greasy. It is also invaluable as an anti-rheumatic treatment.

Neydharting Moor Life Day Cream/Moisturiser
This gentle and light Day Cream/Moisturiser is ideal for all skin types. It is an ideal Day Cream for make-up base and a safe and effective eye cream too.

Neydharting Moor Life Massage Oil

A light oil for daily care of the body skin, foot care, muscle strain, after sports activities and in general ideally suited as a massage oil for full or partial massage. Regular application of the Neydharting Moor Oil improves the blood circulation and tightens the skin. It is very quickly absorbed by the skin.

Neydharting Moor Life Shampoo

The Neydharting Moor Life Shampoo contains all the natural biologically active agents of the Neydharting Healing Moor and is completely free of alkali. It is especially recommended for impaired growth of hair, and hair which has been damaged through harsh permanent waving or dyeing. It is excellent for retarding loss of hair, also for irritation of the scalp and it discourages the formation of dandruff. The Neydharting Moor Shampoo will leave your hair and scalp beautifully clean and your hair manageable, and will give your hair a lovely shine, body and bounce.

Neydharting Moor Life Hair Tonic

Like all Moor products, it works from within, helping to maintain a natural balance. For complete hair and scalp; treatment first wash hair with Moor Shampoo, then massage Moor Hair Tonic into the scalp while your hair is still wet. Do not rinse. Between shampoos, use the Hair Tonic daily on dry hair and scalp for healthy, manageable hair.

Neydharting Moor Life Body Lotion

A recent addition to the Moor Life Beauty range, the body lotion consists of 75% Moor Water in a natural herbal oil carrier, containing all the healing substances derived from hundreds of plants and herbs. This luxurious natural body lotion is delicately perfumed; it stimulates growth of new cells and balances the natural pH factors and skin oil production leaving it refreshed, supple, silky and soft. Apply the lotion liberally after bathing whilst the skin is still moist; truly a wonderful body care lotion and natural moisturiser, moreover, a beautifying and sensual daily experience.

Neydharting Moor Life Toothpaste

A Toothpaste with a difference because it comes from Nature's own Moor, found only at Neydharting in Austria. It preserves the dental enamel, provides a fresh feeling and fresh breath. Gives the teeth a clean white gleam and, due to the natural health giving constituents of the Neydharting Healing Moor, it helps to prevent the development of caries and tooth decay and strengthens the gums. Invaluable for weak and bleeding gums. An ideal supplement to the Moor Mouthwash.

Neydharting Moor Life Mouthwash
Instructions for use:

Simply add a teaspoonful of the Mouthwash to a glass of water, use twice daily to obtain maximum benefit. It helps to prevent mouth odour, pyorrhoea and bleeding of the gums. Excellent for soothing mouth ulcers and sore throats and leaves a refreshing tang to the mouth. Contains all the nutrients of the Neydharting Moor.

"One torch of nature makes the whole world kin"
William Shakespeare

Healing & Cleansing

Premature old age and disease are partly due to the increased accumulation of harmful acids and toxins in the system. This acid and toxic formation is controllable, to just the same extent as old age is controllable. The intolerance of acid in the body is a normal protection for organ function and if we cannot spare enough alkaline from our reserves to neutralise all acids we ultimately die.

All deaths from so called natural causes are merely the end product of a progressive acid and toxic condition. This acid and toxic saturation is progressive almost from the moment of birth through over-feeding, increasing the protein (especially flesh) intake beyond what is necessary for tissue replacement which is the function of protein. Thus when we have reached the point where we can no longer neutralise the acids and toxins present we die, and we are said to have died from natural causes. Such death is always unnatural because it has violated nature's constructive laws and principles.

Once you understand the acid formation and the sources of acid formation you will see that these are self-created. Therefore if understood and not avoided, one is slowly committing suicide by dying from acidosis.

The first of these sources is found in the habit of taking many times as much protein as the body requires for tissue replacement. The building material with which the body is to repair itself consists basically of protein, the most highly acid and toxic forming of all foods. The second cause or source is found in the general consumption of the adulterated, de-alkalised, refined or de-natured foods that are so common, those made from white flour or refined white sugar, acid-forming in themselves and robbed of their own normal alkalinity.

The third source of acid-formation is found in the use of good or bad foods in incompatible mixtures. The fourth source of acid formation is found in the greatly prolonged residence in the colon of fermenting and putrefying food residues, resulting in constipation.

As constipation is caused by rising acidity which lowers function by depleting the alkaline reserves then this fourth source may be regarded as being dependant on the other three, and we can say that all the sources of acid formation in the system are from incorrect nutrition.

The body dies continually and is often reborn, not en masse, but cell by cell, and is it not reasonable to assume that if we recreate the cells of the right materials we will be as young and perfect as when we were first born? Sir William Arbuthnot Lane, the famous English surgeon and doctor, said there is but one disease - a toxic blood circulation.

In combination with a balanced diet including taking daily the Moor Drink and Bath this acid and toxic condition of the organism will in time be eliminated. I recommend twice yearly a full course of Moor Baths and the Moor Drink. Thus by carrying out this healing and cleansing routine all the bodily tissues and structures including the acid alkaline factor will become balanced resulting in a feeling of complete mental and physical renewal. Furthermore, I would advise in order to maintain good health and vitality, that the Moor Drink be taken once daily and a Moor Bath carried out once or twice weekly. This I believe to be a good prophylactic measure against all manner of illness including the prevention and build up of harmful disease producing toxins and acids.

When taken both internally and externally the Moor waters have a detoxifying effect on the whole organism and by virtue of the many normalising and healing agents including important nutrients especially trace minerals and balancing endocrine (hormone) substances the whole psycho-physiological system undergoes a regenerating process.

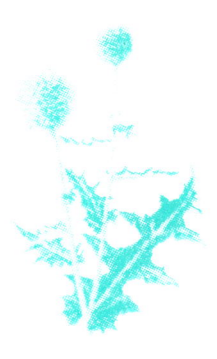

"The atoms in the human body have a corresponding affinity for like atoms in nature"

Head to Toe Health and Beauty The Moor Way

Most people would like to feel they are getting a little younger each day, to experience that their tissues are firming instead of sagging, that ageing spots and lines are beginning to fade, skin elasticity improving, tiredness giving way to natural health and vitality.

Now you can discover new youth, beauty and health by following the Moor Life Health and Beauty Programme in the comfort of your own home, relax and let the deep holistic healing action of the Moor take away the years, the pain and the tiredness. Moor Life is the golden key that unlocks the doors to these priceless assets; moreover subtle and vital radiations encourage the attainment of inner harmony leading to new found vibrant health. You can experience these healing energies flowing throughout your entire organism just like the rising sap from the roots of trees, herbs and plants, travelling throughout their whole biological form giving substance, strength and vitality.

A lovelier skin and more youthful appearance can be yours from Moor Life. It is now time for you to be informed of the Moor's magical secrets. Naturally, it is not possible to reverse the effects of ageing overnight; nature does not work that way. However, given reasonable time and perseverance the thousands of healing herbal and plant substances in perfect balance and harmony will carry out their deep, thorough, healing and regenerating tasks from the skin to the internal organs and glands and from the very depth of the organism to the surface.

Furthermore, the body's own natural sources of energy will be stimulated thus activating it's innate healing powers. You are now about to learn how to put into practice the Moor Head to Toe Health and Beauty Programme and in doing so experience the bountiful gifts of nature through Moor Life.

Health and Beauty Programme

Spring and Autumn, a full course of the Moor Baths, for bathing details refer to pages 27-31. Do not forget the skin brushing routine prior to bathing. The Moor Bouquet Drink taken three times daily during the full bathing programme.

To complement the Moor Bath use the Moor Life Soap so as to restore and maintain the skin's natural pH balance. For women the Cleansing and Toning Lotion can be used daily to refresh and nourish the facial tissues, apply the Face Mask two or three times weekly. See pages 41-45. for skin care routine. The Moor Life Shampoo is unequalled for all types of hair, after which apply the Hair Tonic for that something extra that only Moor Life can give. At night use the Moor Life Face Cream and for day time use the Day Cream Moisturiser.

For really healthy gums and sparkling Teeth brush with Moor Life Toothpaste morning and evening. Spend at least three to five minutes carefully brushing the teeth this will help to prevent dental carries and decay; For the correct way to brush see page 81 on dental care. Should you suffer from gum disorders the Moor Life Mouthwash is soothing and healing.

Women should also carry out the Moor Breast Care

twice weekly during the Spring and Autumn programmes, see Moor Life For Women page 59.

To maintain the improvement in your health, wellbeing and appearance I highly recommend the following programme to be carried out between the Spring and Autumn courses:

Moor Bath	Once or twice weekly
Moor Bouquet	One teaspoon daily
Moor Life Skin Care Programme	Daily - See Page 41-43
Face Mask	Once every seven to ten days
Moor Life Shampoo and Tonic	At least three times weekly
Moor Life Toothpaste - For thorough dental hygiene	am. and pm. daily
Moor Foot Bath	Once weekly - See Page 32
Breast Care Programme	Once every ten days

"Life on this Earth is so short we should all make the most of it by keeping ourselves well and youthful"

Moor, an Elixir of Youth

Man's search for the secret of prolonging human life and vitality began hundreds of years ago. All sorts of strange notions have been tried but to no purpose. Each generation has produced its men of science who have made the quest for a magic elixir of life a special dedication of their time and thought.

Premature old age is one of the greatest tragedies of life. When interest wanes, when fatigue is continual, when minor illnesses become chronic, when food ceases to please, when the former pleasures have all gone, when ambition and enthusiasm are dead, then we are old.

Without health, high spirits, enthusiasm, energy, ambition, enjoyment, undeniably we are old. Without health we are old no matter what term of years, and yet as we shall see premature old age, or sick old age, is not inevitable. Both can be easily and positively avoided.

It is natural for man to be vigorous and well right to the end of his days; it is unnatural for him to be ill. In spite of this fact, however, only 30 per cent of the people of the British Isles die from natural causes, that is to say, from old age. Some 82 per cent die from disease, the other 15 per cent die from accident or misadventure.

The average life span of an animal is five time the time it takes to reach its physical maturity. Man reaches physical maturity at approximately 25 years of age, so it is reasonable to believe that nature intended man to enjoy a life span extending over 125 years.

How tragically we fall short of that is revealed by vital statistics. An animal - dog or horse for instance - lives to at least five times the number of years it takes the animal to mature. Often these animals live until seven times maturity.

Let us consider that divine law as far as man himself is concerned. Man reaches full physical maturity at the age of 21 to 25 years, but does the average man or woman live to the age of a 100 to 125 years?

The average man today can expect to live to be 70, but some doctors think he should live to 150.

The lower animals do much better than man. According to Doctor Edward L. Baltz, a dog is fully grown at 2 years, and lives to an average 12, a cat is fully grown at 1 and lives to 10, a horse fully grown at 4 reaches 25. Therefore, if a man is physically mature at 25, then he should have an average normal life span of 150 years.

Why does man not live proportionately as long as the dog, the horse or other animals? For the simple reason that given the power to think he seems to have lost most of his instinctive powers. He lives and eats by intellect rather than by instinct, and when man traded instinct for intellect he made a disastrous bargain as far as his health was concerned. Instinct would never direct him to adulterated, devitalised foods, starches, artificial sweets and foods high in harmful fats, yet his intellect does. Thus it seems that in the matter of nourishing his body and attaining a ripe old age man fares much worse with his brain than an animal does with its instinctive powers.

The body does not wear out, it is infected out or poisoned out, or starved out, or breaks down through some mineral or vitamin deficiency. If these dangers are deliberately eradicated from your life no evidence exists to show why you should not live to be at least 100.

The search for an elixir of youth has been going on for hundreds of years, yet while modern science still cannot halt the ageing process, there are now more opportunities than ever to remain young and healthy far longer, provided you do not leave it too late.

Our bodies do not want to grow old, our billions of cells wage a continual war against this ageing process. Instead of giving them support in their efforts we over burden them with unnecessary work.

Science informs us that the cells of the human organism can never become old, every minute millions of cells are becoming inert and are eliminated, and new ones are being reproduced.

Give cells the essential nutrients they require and remove before they have time to accumulate and sludge up the body tissues all harmful acids, wastes and toxins; they can be kept alive indefinitely as Dr. Alexis Carrel of the Rockerfeller Institute USA proved by keeping a chicken heart alive for over 30 years. He concluded that "tissue cells are essentially immortal".

I am convinced that with assistance from the Moor the human organism is able to unleash reserves of energy which allows for greater and improved absorption of many vital nutrients which the cells require for their maintenance and also the rapid elimination of ageing waste products, moreover, it does not seem unreasonable to speculate that in the Moor there's a multitude of healing agents in every conceivable form and in perfect synergistic balance which allows the body to remain vital and healthy whatever the age.

"In the future man will use the herbs and plants to regenerate and heal the human body"

(Dr George Crile)

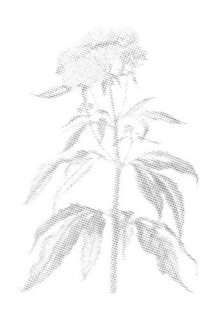

Moor Life for Women

Pregnancy - Motherhood - Babies

A woman's body requires to be beautiful especially during pregnancy and Moor Life can help to achieve this. To obtain the best results possible from regular use of the various Moor Life treatments in pregnancy, a woman should make herself acquainted and knowledgeable about her condition and undertake the necessary measures of "CARE" which consists of four letters C - Circulation, A - Assimilation, R - Relaxation and E - Elimination, all of which are so essential in maintaining health and wellbeing during the nine months of pregnancy. To remain really healthy during this important time is perhaps more essential than at any other period of a woman's life.

The Moor Life Health and Body Care Treatments are nature's healing gifts waiting to give valuable assistance and comfort during pregnancy. Thousands of medicinal plants and herbs which nature through a unique process of maceration has given birth to the rich mud and waters of the Neydharting Healing Moor where in Austria gynaecologist's regularly send their patients.

Numerous health problems often occur during pregnancy for which the Moor Bouquet has proved beneficial, such common disorders as morning sickness, indigestion, constipation, haemorrhoids, sleeplessness, irritability, kidney infections and circulatory problems can all be helped naturally and safely with the Bouquet, furthermore, the various hormone substances contained in the Bouquet assists in contraction of the uterus following the birth.

The Bouquet moreover prepares the body for lactation. Mothers milk is derived directly from her bloodstream. Therefore, whatever she assimilates will be passed directly to her baby through her milk which will contain many nutritional and life sustaining substances from the Bouquet assisting in building up the child's population of essential digestive tract bio-organisms in a ready and active state which the young and growing body requires to develop a vigorous metabolic system, normal eliminative functions, resistance to infections and promotion of both appetite and growth in all parts of the organism which are so necessary in establishing the new arrival on the road to perfect health.

The Moor Life Bath is often referred to as the "Bath of Women" due to its success in infertility. It most certainly helps in conception both before and during to strengthen and balance the organism and following childbirth to repair and heal the body. The bath will relieve spinal, back-muscular and leg pains and tone the skin thus reducing the possibility of both stretch marks and varicose veins.

Moor Life Breast Care Treatment strengthens the breasts and nipples preparing them for breast feeding, firming the breast tissues after birth and lactation and can be used in conditions of breast engorgement and mastitis, applying the treatment in this case daily after which gently work into the breasts the Body Cream.

The Body Cream will help to give the skin complete protection. Apply it to the abdomen and any other areas that require assistance. Used as a hand cream it will prevent chapping and drying and keeps the hands soft and smooth enough to touch and handle the baby.

The Moor Life Soap is ideal for mother and baby's

sensitive skin. It can be used all over the body and is a blessing in skin irritation and nappy rash. Afterwards apply the body cream.

For baby complaints such as stomach cramps, wind, constipation, diarrhoea, teething etc., a small dose of the Bouquet will prove effective. Cradle cap can be treated with the Moor Life Shampoo and Body Cream. For babies with eczema the Moor Bath Soap and Body Cream can bring relief and healing.

The Moor Douche

The Moor Bouquet can be used as a most effective douche for a wide range of tenacious vaginal infections which are so often resistant to all manner of treatments including antibiotics and pessaries.

The Bouquet is both safe and non-irritating used in this way, many beneficial strains of natural bacteria, flora and antibiotics will quickly get to work on irritated, inflamed and infected mucous membranes giving them through nature the opportunity to heal.

Daily douches adding 1-2 teaspoons of the Bouquet to warm filtered water will prove helpful in the majority of cases of vaginitis, thrush, leucorrhea, cervicitis, endocervicitis, etc., in conjunction with daily douching I recommend a course of Moor Baths and the Bouquet which being holistic and constitutional in every way will give to the body the very conditions necessary to heal itself.

Moor Life Breast Care

The Face Mask is also an excellent treatment for breasts that have lost their tissue tone. Through its action on the lymph vessels, waste and toxic matter are eliminated and if used reguarly it will do much to improve the shape, contours and texture of the breasts.

I have advised many ladies who suffer from painful breasts due to lymphatic congestion prior to menstration, also lumpy breasts, providing there is no underlying pathology present, to apply the mask daily a few days before menstruation, also take both the Moor Drink and Bath. The Bath and Drink assists normal hormone functions therefore it can be of considerable assistance to those who suffer from pre-menstrual and menopausal problems.

In treating the breasts with the Face Mask which incidentally contains all the rich goodness of the Moor, is 100 per cent pure and safe. I recommend prior to applying the Mask that the chest and breasts are gently washed in warm water with the Moor Soap. Dilute the Mask by squeezing a small quantity into a cup, add 1-2 teaspoons of water and mix as for facial routine. With a flat make-up brush coated with the Mask reasonably thickly, commencing from the clavicular (collar bones) areas, front of the shoulders and down to the breasts in long sweeping movements taking care to cover the areas well into the sides of the breasts and beneath, the whole of the breasts including the nipples should be covered. Next, apply a couple of large face towels which have been immersed in hot water and squeezed out of excess water, covering each breast, commencing with 3-5 minutes for the first few applications after which increase to no more than 10 minutes. Either remove the Mask with hot cloths or bathing followed by a thorough splashing of the breasts and chest with cold water. After drying gently, massage a little Moor Life Face cream into the breasts.

For all women who are desirous of a good bust line I thoroughly recommend this treatment which can be carried out weekly for life.

Scar tissue and stretch marks on the abdomen can alsso be improved with the Mask treatment, applying in a similar manner.

The Menopause

Women who are entering and going through the menopause with its accompanying array of unpleasant symptoms can be considerably helped by Moor Life on account of the valuable wealth of natural nutritional and hormone sub stances it contains.

The Moor Bath and Bouquet can prove to be of immense value in cases of hot flushes and sweats, lethargy, depression, insomnia, aches and pains, headaches, hair and skin changes, loss of self esteem and confidence, vaginal and urinary symptoms etc.

I recommend full courses of the Bath and Bouquet at regular intervals including sitz bathing for local pelvic disorders. The Moor Life Skin and Hair Care routine will help with premature hair loss and ageing and wrinkling of the tissues. To improve and maintain a good bust line the Moor Breast Care routine can be carried out regularly. In cases of vaginal dryness and discomfort the Moor Life Body Cream is most effective.

Finally, all Moor Life products are absolutely safe, in fact they are literally safe enough to be eaten. They stand alone in the world as being the only range of internal and external treatments that are "NATURE'S VERY OWN" and can at all times and under all conditions be trusted upon. It has been said that Moor Life Cream is the first aid you need in the the house, Moor Life Bouquet (Drink) is the doctor you need in the house!

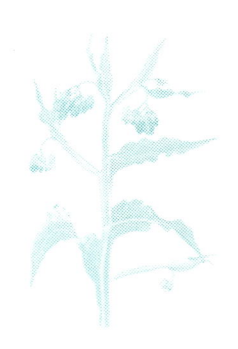

The Moor for Sportsmen and Women

Nearly every one who participates in sports, either in actual competition or training, will suffer at some time from an injury. This can range from bruising or muscle stiffness to injuries such as strained or torn tendons, ligaments, and muscles, stress fractures and broken bones.

Whatever the injury the Moor Life Treatments can help in getting back to normal more quickly than would otherwise be possible.

Let me examine some of the possible injuries and detail the recommended Moor Life Treatment for the particular condition in question.

Muscular stiffness and soreness: The important point here is to improve and increase the local blood supply to the tissues affected. This can be achieved by applications of Moor Compresses to the muscles after which massaging either the Body Cream or Massage Oil into the troublesome area. Alternatively soak in a Moor Life Bath resting after wards.

Bruising: The main effects of bruising are swelling and inflammation which impairs the circulation thus preventing cells from receiving an adequate supply of oxygen. To the bruised and surrounding area apply a Moor Compress, also Moor Life Baths can be of considerable use. Do not massage the area however, gently cover the bruised tissues with the Moor Life Body Cream.

Damaged tendons and ligaments can be treated with Compresses after which applying the Moor Life Body Cream or Massage Oil.

Should a fracture or broken bone occur urgent hospital treatment is necessary. Once the parts have healed, the Moor will play an important part in speeding full recovery. In such cases a course of Moor Life Baths, also use of the Massage Oil will prove efficacious.

As a former long distance and marathon runner I can vouch for the Moor's speedy healing efficacy. On many occasions during long training runs and competing in full marathons I sustained all manner of muscle, tendon and joint strains which the Moor Life Bath, Body Cream and Massage Oil took care of. My recovery from the effects of marathon running were extremely quick provided afterwards I took a full Moor Life Bath. During the 1982 Stockholm Marathon I suffered from a badly strained Achilles tendon which after completing the gruelling twenty-six miles I could barely walk. Fortunately I had in my travelling bag the Moor Body Cream. After hot and cold applications under the shower I generously worked into the painful area the Moor Life Cream. By the following morning, much to my amazement and delight I was able to walk almost normally which enabled me to make the journey home in reasonable comfort. After training and competitions the Moor Life Bath will quickly remove fatigue products from the body as I have personally proved.

No sportsman or woman should be without the invaluable healing assets of the Neydharting Moor. Those who experience aches and pains after gardening or other active pursuits, also manual workers, will find relief with Moor Life.

Colon Health

The Colon

The colon is the large, lower bowel. It is five feet long but is crowded into a very small space. It starts in the lower right side, goes straight upward to the liver, across to the spleen under the lower left ribs, then down to the floor of the pelvis where it empties. It is a series of many pouches and convolutions where refuse finds easy stoppage. Medicines and enemas only empty the lower twelve inches of it, leaving quantities of poisonous debris to cling to the lining of the remaining four feet and cause absorption of these poisons in to the circulation of the body.

SLOW ELIMINATION MEANS SLOW DECAY OF MIND AND BODY

Just to the degree that elimination is retarded the whole system becomes poisoned, mind and body become indolent, efficiency lessens, disease takes root, and the mind and body decay. Primitive people on a high roughage diet store their faecal matter only for less than 18 hours in the colon. The low roughage, highly concentrated foods of the typical Western diet take from 72 hours to 6 days to pass out of the body and the poisons of decay are absorbed into the body. As no system can perpetually bear the ravages of self-poisoning, inadequate elimination means inferior health and a shorter life.

Elimination of body generated toxic and waste products occurs only through the skin, the lungs and kidneys. When one of these eliminative channels becomes retarded or inactive from any cause, the other organs of elimination are handicapped and slowed up by the increased burden forced upon them. Hence, it is frequently found that the toxic refuse in the bowels is one to ten days late in passing out, which means that the poisons which should have been eliminated are reabsorbed and taken back into the circulation.

CONSTIPATION CAUSES MANY AILMENTS

Babies, animals and primitive people will eliminate, that is, empty their bowel after each meal. This is normal. All else is constipation. The bowels either fail to move at all without artificial assistance, or force out today that which should have been eliminated one to ten days ago. As the kidneys and other eliminative channels are unable to dispose of the refuse in the bowels the poisons remain in the body to cause or help cause such conditions as liver disease, frequent colds, asthma, skin problems, circulatory diseases, high blood pressure, bladder trouble, female problems, prostate trouble, cancer of the colon or rectum, colitis, diverticulitis, appendicitis, hemorrhoids, varicose veins, listlessness, head aches, sleepnessness and many others including cancer.

CATHARTICS, LAXATIVES AND ENEMAS

While cathartics and laxatives have been a blessing to

civilized people, continual use of them is injurious to the system. It is a fact that they are irritating and therefore able to produce permanent damage, which makes the bowels struggle to expel them quickly. Enemas are not efficient, and work aginst nature. They normally are only effective on the lowest part of the bowel and the amount of water retained during the application causes distention of the lower colon which can result in damage. It is also possible to rupture the bowel under certain conditions.

WHY MOOR COLON THERAPY IS EFFECTIVE AND SAFE

WHEN CORRECTLY GIVEN, colon therapy removes quickly all the toxic debris and poisons from the entire colon and frequently produces permanent relief from stubborn constipation, thus helping to relieve the conditions arising from poor elimination; it assists in the purification of the blood and in the elimination of poisons from the system. It does not dilate or irritate the colon. The water flows out at the same rate it flows in. Although many gallons of water are used in each treatment, it is painless and not unpleasant. There is no exposure and no embarrassment. The number of treatments depends on the patient's condition, age and how long it has existed. An occasional irrigation after the old trouble is cleared up helps to maintain good health. Furthermore, the Moor contains an abundance of natural friendly flora and bacteria including antibiotics, harmful toxins and pathogenicmicro-organisms living within the colon will be quickly destroyed, also many nutritious substances and enzymes are absorbed through the bowels mucous membranes providing strength and tone resulting in improved peristalsis allows the colon to eliminate old impacted faecial materials, the Moor Bouquet, therefore, is an effective and natural means of achieving colon cleanliness and health.

As recommended by Professor Stober, Neydharting Moor, that "blessing in brown", is added to the water especially for the humic acids it contains, which are inflammation-inhibitive. The other healing substances in the rich Moor Bouquet all make their characteristic contributions.

COMMON OBJECTIONS

1. *It is not natural* - but neither is an obstructed or engorged colon natural. Any sickness is unnatural and until a system can be restored to its natural condition we must assist nature and remove impurities from the system.

2. *It is debillitating* - Hundreds of people have attested to the contrary. Personal experience is the only valued fact.

3. *It causes the intestines to become weakened and dependent on this unnatural method* - At least 50% of the people in so-called civilized countries are slaves to laxatives. This is habit forming and dangerous as explained above: Flushing the colon does not cause weakness of the intestines. Due to restored health, the intestines are also restored and improved in tone, and will carry on their functions unaided. Most patients resume normal bowel functions, some even after 30 years of laxative dependency.

4. *Repeated use of the colon therapy will stretch and permanently distend the colon* - This is opposed to physiological law. Repeated flexion and extension of an arm, for

instance, will strengthen its muscles, not cause them to lose their ability to contract, and so do the muscles of the colon get stronger by exercise.

5. *It operates against peristalsis* - Not true. When treating a patient, normal peristaltic action is encouraged.

6. *Washing of the interior surface of the colon is injurious since it washes away the natural lubricants* - Does bathing the external surface of the body prevent further excretions of the skin? Does bathing of the eye destroy the function of the lacrimal glands? Does washing of the mouth or drinking fluids prevent any further secretion of saliva or of stomach juices? If washing away of a secretion would destroy the power of secreting glands, then human existence would indeed be brief.

Colon Cleansing - Important to Total Health

As seen by the above, todays modern lifestyle is responsible for premature ageing, and 80% of the population suffer from some form of constipation. Most people don't realize it or recognize it. Colon cleansing through colon therapy is a safe, sensible way to keep healthy or it can be used as an aid in the regaining of health. Physicians at the Royal Society in Great Britain discussed problems relating to "alimentary toxemia." The conclusions reached after research and the study of case histories was that alimentary toxemia was often the beginning of serious disease and disorders throughout the body.

EVACUATION AFTER EVERY MEAL

A common complaint from colon therapists is: "Patients thank us for the relief and then return to the way of life that caused the condition. " To avoid recurrence of the trouble you should follow a sensible diet which includes plenty of natural fibre, fruits and vegetables. If you feel that an "evacuation after every meal" is too much for you to aim for, at least cultivate the habit of having an evacuation every morning and evening. For that endeavour, do NOT take purgatives, do NOT sit down and try to force your colon. The proper method is psychological and gentle, but effective, if you persist. They are "imagine" and "expect". The only wilforce you have to use is to visit the toilet twice a day, whatever happens. Finally I would like to see all those who practice Colonic Irrigation Therapy to consider and see for themselves the enormous advantages that the Moor Bouquet has over other herbal agents in colon cleansing and maintenance.

"Keep your bowel and blood stream clean and you need fear no disease"

Dr Henry Lindlahr

Moor Life Massage

Massage is a most healing and pleasurable experience. It is difficult to overstate the satisfaction of massage because the therapeutic benefits are so numerous. Beside the many physical effects there are almost, if not more, psycho logical ones.

Massage is one of the oldest forms of healing known to many civilizations. In 400 BC. Hippocrates, known as the "Father of all Healing ", employed massage to treat his patients. Massage remains an effective drugless therapy; there are very few parts of the body which do not respond or benefit from it.

Massage activates the flow of lymphatic fluids; blood circulation is enhanced both venous and arterial; skin and muscle tone are improved, digestion and elimination is speeded up; endocrine (hormone) functions are stimulated, fatigue products are cleared away. Regular massage stimu lates and also relaxes the whole nervous system.

Massage has a profound effect on stress related conditions. Many doctors believe that massage can take the place of psychotherapy treatment. The real benefit of massage is a general feeling of relaxation and well being. A full body massage soothes, stimulates and enlivens the whole body especially if the Moor Life Massage Oil is used as it contains all the natural healing constituents of over 1,000 herbs and plants from the Neydharting Healing Moor blended with pure and natural plant oils.

For general massage use, add 15 to 20 drops to a pure carrier oil such as almond. This will produce a massage oil of considerable healing potential. Prior to use the oil should be gently heated so as to allow improved absorption by the skin. The Moor Life Massage Oil is unequalled in its healing effects. I usually use it after osteopathic manipulation as it compliments the manipulative work thus speeding up the healing process.

Massage Suggestions

Contra-indications; fever, bruises, tumours, skin disorders, thrombosis, phlebitis, varicose and sensitive veins, open sores, wounds, infections, fractures, acute stomach disorders, menstruation, complications in pregnancy, recent surgical scars, on a full stomach.

Massage in a warm room using towels to cover the areas that are not being treated. Since the skin is going to receive treatment it would be beneficial to take a warm bath or shower using the Moor Life Soap. The most effective massage is given on a massage couch or plinth, however, several blankets over a sleeping bag or large cushions placed on the floor is adequate, a sheet should cover the blankets for the recipients comfort, also have a pillow or two nearby to place under the knees and head. Maintain a consistent and even rhythm throughout. Jerky movements are to be avoided, always balance the movements equally to both sides of the body. Relaxing music can be helpful to induce relaxation in the recipient and as an aid for the operator's hands to work to.

Make sure that the hands are warm and nails short. The oil to be used must be poured onto the palms and rubbed into the hands not directly onto the recipient's body.

The Moor Natures Healing Miracle

Effleurage

Effleurage

Effleurage

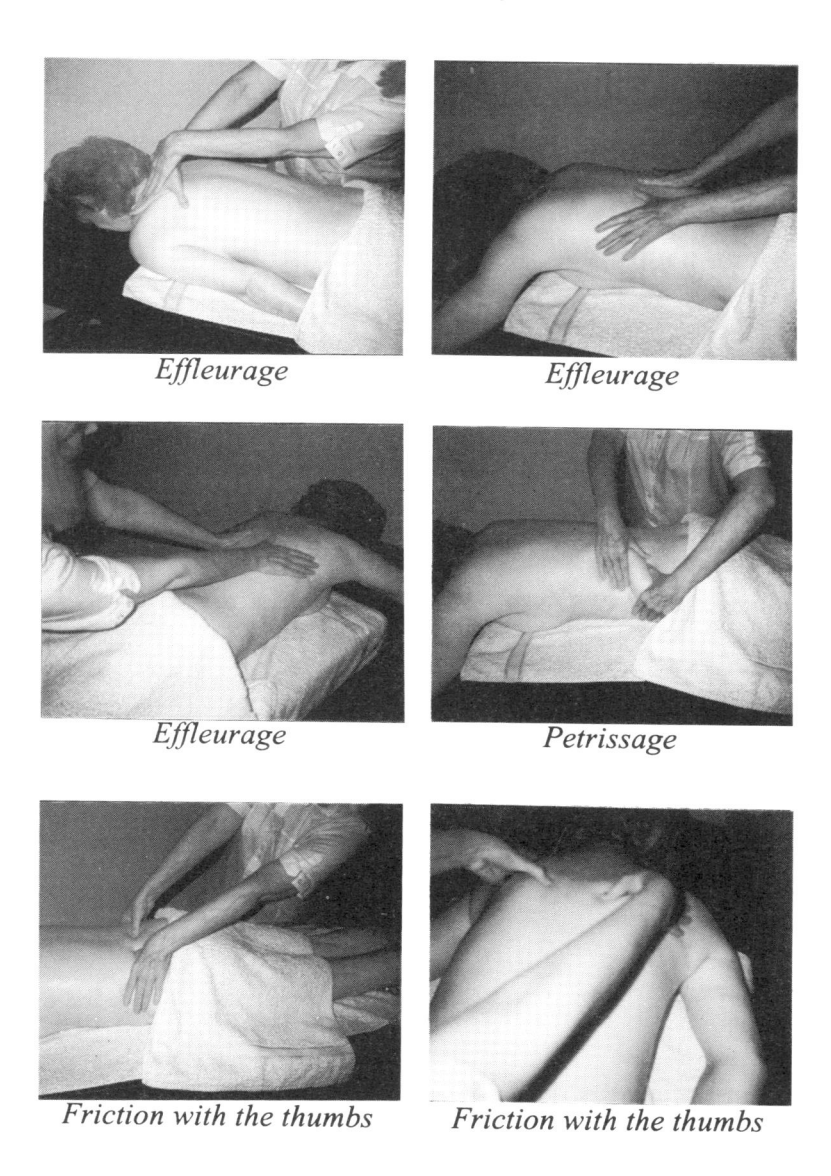

Petrissage

Friction with the thumbs

Friction with the thumbs

In order to become proficient in massage it is necessary to attend classes, proper massage cannot be learnt from the printed word, however, the following movements are reasonably simple to carry out. They can be used individually or combined with others of your own choice. The main purpose of this massage routine is to allow the healing properties of the Moor Life Massage Oil thorough absorption into the blood vessels of the skin from where it has a beneficial and healing effect on the internal organs and tissues.

Basic Movements

Effleurage; gently but firmly glide the hands with long even strokes over the surface of the body, the direction is towards the heart, this movement can be used all over the body. The hands should at all times remain in contact with the body moulding them to whatever part is being treated. Apply a deep pressure towards the heart and light contact on the downward movement.

With the recipient lying face down commence at the feet . . . to the calves . . . knees . . . thighs . . . hips . . . and then over the back to the neck. After finishing effleurage commence picking up and rolling the tissues like kneading dough. Friction consists of a small circular movement carried out with the pads of the thumbs, fingers and heel of the hand. Finish off with effleurage then have the recipient on their back with a pillow under the knees and head commencing with effleurage from toes to lower leg . . . knee . . . thigh . . . groin. Fingers to arms . . . shoulders . . . sides of abdomen . . . to armpits . . . lower chest round breasts to shoulders. Petrissage and friction follows effleurage in the same manner as for the back, ending with effleurage.

The abdomen receives effleurage commencing at the

navel in a clockwise direction in ever increasing circles after which petrissage, finishing off with effleurage. Cover the recipient with a large towel and quietly leave him/her to relax so as to absorb the deep healing effects of the treatment.

Should you receive regular massage treatment from a professional therapist, introduce him/her to the Moor Life Massage Oil. I am sure your practitioner will be pleasantly surprised with the results, moreover, the deep healing effect of the Oil will considerable assist practitioners of massage, osteopathy, acupuncture, reflexology, aromatherapy, ma nipulation and chiropody in their healing work.

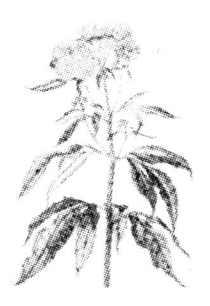

"Human hands are Natures perfect tools for healing"

Hair, Scalp, Dental, Hand Care

The human head of hair is a most remarkable product of the body. Like nails which have a close chemical affinity with it, hair grows many times faster than other body cells. Both the hair and nails could be described as the barometer or indicator of the general state of health.

One single hair has a lifespan of five years in a person of good health. It takes approximately 4 years for one hair to grow and develop, and between 2-4 weeks for degradation at the end of which the hair finally dies and falls out.

Human hair grows a little over 1cm a month. In the summer months and warmer periods it grows very much faster than in the winter. It is normal for the head to lose approximately 50 hairs each day and somewhat more during spring and autumn. Therefore it is no reason to be concerned over this quite natural and necessary process. Very few people realise that the hair on the back of the head is used by the body for elimination of acids and toxins via the kidneys and may tend to become thicker or even undergo a straw like appearance as highly toxic waste is allowed to accumulate in the organism.

The first things to do when the hair lacks lustre, vitality and liveliness is to stop abusing it and starving it of nourishment. Bleaching, perming, the use of dryers and harsh combing and brushing can over a period of time result in lost vitality and lustre. One sign above all others is abnormal hair loss; as previously explained a healthy scalp continually does shed a percentage of its hair but it is constantly replaced.

Scientific investigation has revealed that women with normal thyroid functions have beautiful hair. Sadly, it has been medically established that women who suffer thyroid imbalances experience considerable hair problems including loss. When the thyroid is overactive hair loss can be somewhat high either over the scalp in general or in particular areas, hair on examination will be found to be abnormally thin and break easily. Underactivity of the thyroid produces brittleness and dryness with resultant all over hair loss.

Improvement in hair health must commence from the inside of the body. It makes very little difference whatever is directly applied, hairs can grow only from the roots. It is particularly for reversing the effects of damage caused by chemicals used in perms, lotions, colorants, also the use of metal combs and dryers which deposit an electrostatic charge attracting dirt and foreign particles that Moor Life Hair Care has no equal. Due to the unique herbs and substances it contains, Moor Life will in a comparatively short period of time help to repair damaged hair.

Treatment is both internal and external. The Bouquet will help to correct various metabolic and other imbalances and have a cleansing effect on the organism. Three doses are recommended daily over a period of several weeks. The Moor Life Shampoo and Hair Tonic should be used every other day, its action is to penetrate the scalp acting on the very centres of hair life, the roots.

Moor Life Hair Care will stimulate head and scalp circulation resulting in increased life giving lymph flow, thus enabling hair in its entirety to be nourished, revitalised and strengthened. Furthermore, this treatment performs the necessary function of supplying important substances to the hair roots therefore giving protection to the hair shafts which prevents irritation and dandruff, at the same time removing grease and other injurious foreign bodies from the scalp and finally, it gives body and strength to fine hair restoring vitality and lustre to hair whether normal, dry, brittle or damaged.

Dental Health

Firstly it is recommended that the ideal toothbrush consists of rounded nylon bristles which are soft. The correct way to brush is to place the ends of the bristles into the crevices between the teeth using gentle pressure allowing the bristles to reach the gums, next wiggle the brush backwards and forwards applying very short strokes, this technique will assist in dislodging fine particles of plaque from the crevices which is one of the major factors in periodontal disease. Each tooth should be treated in the same manner top and bottom. The teeth consist of five surfaces, front, top, back and two sides which to remain healthy and free of plaque must be methodically cleaned preferably after each meal. It will be found efficacious to apply very short strokes of a vibrational nature which cleans the teeth more thoroughly than the usual method. As well as dislodging plaque this brushing technique will at the same time remove harmful bacterial deposits that accumulate daily. By brushing in this manner using the Moor Life Toothpaste and rinsing with the Mouthwash the teeth should remain plaque free and the gums healthy, the whole procedure taking approximately five minutes, time well spent in maintaining good dental hygiene and health.

Care of the Hands

The hands form a special relationship with the body in reaching out and feeling the environment around us, being sensory organs of locomotion they convey all manner of sensory signals through the nervous system to various parts of the body, furthermore, the human body consists of subtle electro-magnetic fields with electro-magnetic energy flowing through and around it finishing up in the feet and hands which reflexologists refer to as reflex points or zones.

These reflex points have a direct influence and relationship with both our internal and external physiology, every organ, gland or part of the body has an appropriate zone or reflex point on the feet and hands which if stimulated can exert a most beneficial and healing reaction on the organ or part in question.

As the Moor Foot Bath stimulates the reflex points of the feet benefiting the whole body, the Moor Treatment for the Hands will likewise have a beneficial and stimulative action on the whole physiology.

Commence treatment by washing the hands in warm water using the Moor Soap; really work a good lather up spending sufficient time in working the resultant lather well into both hands including the fingers, thumbs and nails after which rinse in cold water and dry. Finally, using the Body Cream, thoroughly massage into both hands including the fingers and thumbs spending approximately 5 minutes on each hand which will leave them feeling soft, smooth and supple.

Animals - Pets - Plants - Gardens

Not only can the Moor help suffering mankind, it can also prove efficacious in a wide range of diseases that afflict animals. Moor Treatment can be extremely successful in the restoration and maintenance of health in both domestic and farm animals including horses. All creatures are more in touch with nature than the majority of human beings. Their innate instincts guide them in times of illness and injury to herbs, healing plants and waters.

As a result of scientific findings in veterinary medicine on the Moor, a new field of application has been opened up in the treatment of animals. With this purpose in mind, approximately 10 years ago, Neydharting Moor Scientists successfully developed and produced two unique products, namely, Moor Harvest for Animals and Pets and Wild Forage for Horses, both of these feeding supplements are 100 % natural and safe.

Moor Harvest and Wild Forage consist of natural extracts from a variety of over a thousand different wild flowers, plants, grasses and herbs all naturally preserved over thousands of years in the Neydharting Moor. Grazing animals such as horses and cattle will receive from Moor supplementation a wealth of nutritional materials including vitamins, minerals, trace minerals, amino acids, natural antibiotics and others that they would ingest, if grazing naturally in the wild.

Veterinary practitioners in Austria and several other countries have recorded a great number of proven successes with Moor Harvest when prescribed to farm animals.

Professor A Senze of Poland undertook experiments with Moor Harvest in cases of mastitis in cows; out of 50 cases involved, a positive result was obtained in 47 cows. An old cow quite suddenly yielded an increase in her milk production from 4 litres to 12 litres a day after being given Moor Harvest.

Observations made on individual species of animals revealed a remarkable success rate after almost immediate application of the Moor Harvest supplement; sickly and weak animals after a few days showed improved appetite for food and became healthy and vigorous once more.

During feeding experiments it was observed in veterinary clinics and university hospitals for animals that the animals which were given Moor Harvest grew faster and became heavier than those who did not receive supplementation.

Further studies and experiments with veterinary practitioners revealed that during wide-spread foot and mouth disease animals prescribed the Moor Supplement showed increased resistance to the disease, whilst animals suffering from the disease did not lose their appetite when prescribed the supplement because the inflamed mucous vesicles in the mouth caused by the disease became less inflamed and painful. Furthermore, cattle who regularly received Moor Harvest were less likely to be afflicted with viral diseases in general.

A report of interest by Dr. Josef Arth, in respect to the prophylactic treatment of honey bees with the Moor Drink revealed that Nosema, a particularly serious disease affecting bees, was prevented by adding a quantity of Moor Drink to the bees' drinking water, a second drink of pure water was made available, however all the bees preferred the Moor Drink avoiding the pure water, which quite clearly illustrates the innate intelligence at work.

Domestic dogs and cats who suffer from arthritis, rheumatism, kidney disorders, skin problems, gastro-intestinal complaints, including diarrhoea, show a remarkable improvement and in many cases a complete cure following treatment with the Moor Drink. Pregnant and whelping bitches, poorly out of condition and old animals respond well to the health and tonic effects of Moor Harvest.

Pets who suffer from skin irritations, bites, wounds, sores, cracked pads, etc., can be treated with the Moor Life Body Cream.

Moor Harvest is suitable for all animals including birds, both in times of sickness and as a prophylactic measure against illness. Because of its inflammation inhibiting, detoxifying and appetite promoting properties "Moor Harvest" is nature's remedy for a diversity of diseases that animals including our beloved pets are prone to.

Wild Forage is used in the treatment of Horses, Foals and Ponies. It is prescribed for peak performance, stamina, fertility, promotion of healthy growth and weight gains, prevention of digestive disorders, excess acid etc.

University Professor - Dr G Del Seppia, Florence, Italy reported in his article 'Moor Therapy for Horses' published in 'Austrian Moor Research' as follows:

"For many years I have been using WILD FORAGE, treating Race Horses with considerable success. Underfed, weak and exhausted horses were given 20 - 30ml per day. This usually restored appetites within 3-4 days and it had a normalising effect on the digestive function. The horses became lively and strong again quickly"

University Lecturers Drs. Vet M Kostner and P Silbert. Graz, Austria authors of 'Oral Treatment for Horses' which was publicised in 'Vienna Veterinary Monthly' - excerpts as follows:

"With WILD FORAGE we are able to improve illnesses in Horses which have pathogenetic connections with illnesses of the stomach and intestinal tracts, also some skin disorders, in much the same way as illnesses of the stomach and intestinal tracts themselves. Most horses accept WILD FORAGE spontaneously as it is tasteless and odourless".

Moor Compresses are indicated for all conditions for which hot dressings or hot compresses are normally administered, e.g. inflammation of tendon sheaths, joints, arthritis, myositis etc.

List of Universities that have conducted research work into the Neydharting "Moor Harvest natural feed supplement for all animals:

Austria	:	Veterinary Institutes of Vienna Graz and Innsbruck.
Finland	:	Helsinki University.
Germany	:	Universities of Bremen & Hanover, Munich Veterinary Institute.
Hungary	:	Universities of Budapest, Helikon and Keszthely.

Italy	:	Universities of Florence, Milan Pavia, Rome, Turin.
Poland	:	Agricultural College of Wroclaw.
United Kingdom	:	University of Cambridge.

On conclusion, I wholeheartedly recommend the reader who raises and keeps animals and has the welfare of animals at heart to avail themselves of the enormous healing potential of Moor Harvest and Wild Forage for since the days of old it has been observed that sick or injured animals wallowed in and drank the dark healing waters of the Neydharting Moor.

"Nature created the Moor
As a healing place
Not just for man for
Since the world began
Lame and sick animals have come
To drink it's waters and
Feed upon it's herbs
Gone on their way, restored
Chosen by god to show
A sick mankind the way to perfect health
Thanks be to Mother Nature her Animals and the Moor".

B. Ditcher

Flora-Moor for Plants and Gardens

Flora-Moor consists of natural plant substances derived

from thousands of different herbs, plants, grasses and flowers that has taken nature many thousands of years to form in the Neydharting Moor. Being a complete organic plant food Flora-Moor can be used on indoor and outdoor plants, flowers, vegetables and fruit. Besides supplying hundreds of nutrients in a balanced form Flora-Moor increases the transportation of vital energy from the Moor's various plant substances to plants and soil.

Regular use of Flora-Moor on plants, vegetables, roses, flowers, etc., can result in much sturdier growth, healthier and heavier blooms, flowers also increase in numbers and take on a more colourful appearance. Furthermore insecticides, fungicides and other damaging toxic chemicals become increasingly unnecessary as a result of plants improved resistance to diseases including invasion from insect pests etc. I have noticed the soil around Flora-Moor treated plants develop a richness and darkness which is so reminiscent of the Moor's goodness and vitality, for this reason Flora-Moor makes an ideal natural soil conditioner.

Observations by scientists at the Moor Research Institute have shown oat seedlings when sprayed with dilute Moor grew many times faster than was usual. Also sickly and weak trees given the Moor solution recovered their vigour quickly.

For the enrichment of compost Flora-Moor is excellent. By watering each layer of the heap with diluted Flora-Moor a richer organic humus is produced.

Flora-Moor can be used on any kind of plants and is ideally applied whilst watering in the normal way. Furthermore, used as a foliar spray on leaves and branches it will improve both condition and resistance to disease. Flora-Moor is kind on the environment correcting and redressing the imbalances that toxic chemicals cause. It's considerable versatility is a great asset to the organic gardener. By using Flora-Moor we are giving back to nature in perfect balance and harmony all the goodness that only nature herself can supply. Finally, Flora-Moor is 100 % Natural and Organic, is not harmful to children, pets or wildlife and is 100 % Environmentally Friendly.

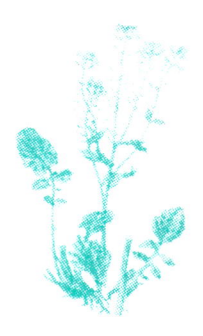

"All the goodness is as the plants and herbs of nature"

Life Energy Fields

"Energy is a Living Force which emanates from Consciousness"....

Within the human organism is a subtle yet dynamic electro-chemical source of healing which given the correct stimulus creates powerful energy fields that exert healing impressions to the organic cellular structures of the body.

Science is aware that all living organisms are surrounded and permeated by subtle Life Energy Fields which can be seen in beautiful colours and patterns as Kirlian Photography so well demonstrates. Should this flow of Life Energy become weakened or blocked in any way its control over the many cells relating to the respective organism diminishes resulting in cellular disharmony and degradation.

Life is basically an energy experience, all human interactions as well as physiological functions are purely vibrational in nature.

On the human physical level the slowing down or blocking of energy flow through the various organs and other physiological structures will cause disharmony and imbalance within the corresponding organs and tissues thus ultimately resulting in physiological dysfunction and finally disease. Disease, therefore, can be said to be the end result of interrupted and poor subtle energy flow through areas of the body's physiology.

Taken that the Moor functions on all energy levels

including the spiritual it can be said that its subtle energy radiations have the power to stimulate the body's own electro-chemical charges into healing the physiology.

I am indebted to Nigel Garion-Hutchings for his most excellent Kirlian Photographs taken from small samples of the Moor Bathing Liquid, Drink and Massage Oil his valued observations and report are as follows:

Kirlian electro-photography and the Moor.

Kirlian electro-photography is based upon observations of phenomenon known as the corona discharge which appears around objects that are put into high-frequency electrical fields. Semyon Kirlian discovered that the corona discharge patterns reveal significant information pertaining to the hidden energy dynamics of the substance photographed. It is significant that devitalised substance gives off a much duller and reduced corona discharge than does vital and dynamic substance.

The Moor samples show concentrated corona discharges, (energy field) that emanate very strongly indeed. Considering that dead or devitalised substances produce little if any corona discharge it would seem reasonable to surmise that the Moor samples are in the dynamic class. This would confirm that which has been reported by those who have benefited from using the Moor.

Of the samples photographed the pure Moor Bathing Liquid has an obviously stronger corona disharge than the drink. The massage oil which has Moor in it also shows a strong field yet is more contained and has finer emanations. The Moor Drink shows the same characteristics of the pure sample (notice how it spreads beyond the initial concentrated energy field) yet is obviously not as strong in comparison.

Kirlian photographs were also taken of the samples in a glass petrie dish. The samples covered the entire bottom of the dish yet the energy fields took on an almost animated three dimensional character. The corona discharges have similar characteristic to the previous samples, which were photographed in thin polythene, yet appear more contained. In the glass dish the pure Moor energy field seems a little brighter than the drink and has a slightly stronger corona while the oil continues to have a finer and reduced corona. In all cases there is an aliveness and dynamic quality that suggests that this is indeed a vital substance.

Nigel Garion-Hutchings is a practising Homoeopath, metaphysical teacher and life counsellor. He has been working with Kirlian photography since the seventies and is considered a leading authority in this field. Over the last 17 years he has held seminars and courses on Homoeopathy and Kirlian electro-photography in this country and abroad. He is co-author of the best selling book "The Concise Guide To Homoeopathy" published by Element and is currently writing another on Kirlian photography and the healing power of crystals, herbs and symbols, which is due for publication in 1994.

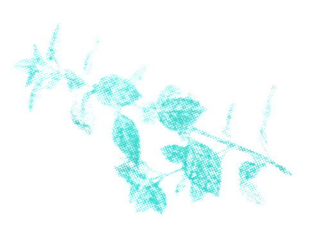

"Every element of the planet is within the human body we are the microcosm within a macrocosm"

Scientific and Medical Opinions Including Reports

Dr. Kaiser, University Professor, Vienna. The Clinic of the University continuously conducted investigations of the duodenal secretion under the treatment with Neydharting moor drink which demonstrated after some days that fixed cultures showed an essential decline of the pathogenic germs. The leucocytes (colourless blood corpuscles) increased quickly and the values normalized themselves by the treatment with Neydharting moor drink already after some days.

Dr. J. Kowarschik, Privy Councillor, University Professor, Vienna. Austria:
"... As far as the quality of the Neydharting moor earth is concerned, I must agree that it is a most excellent one. It is not surpassed by any other Moor Spa of Austria".

Dr. Burghard Breitner, University Professor, Privy Councillor, President of the Austrian Red Cross Society and Head of the Surgical Clinic of the University of Innsbruck, Tyrol, Austria:
"... A noteworthy improvement took place after the Neydharting moor Schwebstoff cure (subjectively as well as objectively."

Professor Dr. Kotschau, Bad Harzburg, Germany:
"But this moor-bouquet does not act in this way that every disease would get its treatment by a specific remedy

occuring in the bouquet, but it acts as a whole complex upon the organism and its powers of defence and healing..."

Dr. V. Klare, Superior Medical Officer, and Dr. W. Chitil, Vienna, Austria:

"... The favourable influence of the moor bath upon inflammatory diseases as well as upon hypoplasia of the female genital tract has been sufficiently known for a long time. This good therapeutical effect cannot come about just by a thermal or mechanical effect of the moor bath, but by its chemical action. Long ago Professor Kowarschik has clearly referred to the circumstance that the essential effect of the moor bath must be a chemical one. He stated that the thermal effect is not characteristic in any way, and practically could be replaced by a water bath and that the mechanical effect of the moor bath is therapeutically insignificant and that the hindrance of the movement of the body as well as of the respiration (of the person bathing in the moor *pulp*) may even be regarded as a disadvantage.

"Thus, the chemical factors undoubtedly play an essential role in the effect of the moor bath, especially since the favourable effect of the moor bath upon rheumatic diseases with a disordered hormonal balance cannot be explained solely by the local, thermal and mechanical components; neither by the stress-effect eventually resulting therefrom. These effects, which we can obtain also by many other methods of treatment, but nevertheless, we thereby cannot attain these favourable results of treatment. Consequently, chemical substances must get into the blood vessels via the skin...

"During this Congress competent scientists have delivered interesting and valuable reports relative to the kind and composition of these chemical substances. We are chiefly interested in the endocrinely influenced rheumatic diseases, especially in the *estrogenoid* substances. These substances originated from the *Fruchtstande* (the inflorescences after the frutification) of the plants submerged in the moor and seem to have an effect similar to the follicle hormone. They may not only have the favourable therapeutic effect in various gynaecological diseases, for instance, genital hypoplasia, sterility, etc., but may also have an essential therapeutic effect by a direct or indirect action upon the hormonal household of the endocrinely disordered rheumatic diseases. This conclusion urgently crowds into one's mind..."

Donawitz Smelting Works, Administration of the Sick Fund:
"Neydharting drinking cures have shown excellent results."

Dr. Heinrich di Gaspero, University Professor, Graz, Austria:
"In the extensive projects of moor research, the physio-chemical foundation as well as the biological effects on the whole organism in the healthy and diseased, were taken into consideration. At this point I wish to mention the biological-functions of the skin.... I am convinced that particularly the Neydharting moor products are able to produce lasting dermal reactions, which result in penetrative effects on the whole organism via alteration of the skin functions...."

Dr. Rheinhold Buller, University Professor, Head of the Ambulatory Clinic of the General Hospitals of the City of Vienna, Austria:
"...In the Third Medical Department Moor from

Neydharting was tried in various concentrations for the treatment of stomach diseases. In this treatment there were included ordinary catarrhs, as well as people suffering from ulcers.... The Neydharting moor is harmless also when taken orally...."

Medical Department of the State Hospital, Graz, Austria; Head: Dr. Stefan Greif, University Professor:
"We use the Neydharting moor drink cure. This cure has turned out well, indeed, in all kinds of gastritis, duodenitis, as well as in the various ulcers of the stomach and duodenum. It was striking that the burdensome pains disappeared in almost all cases in a short time after the beginning of the cure... We could not determine attendant phenomena of any detrimental kind."

General Public Hospital of the State of Carinthia, First Medical Department, Klagenfurt, Austria; Director: Dr. Ignaz Kallus, Privy Councillor, Superior Medical Officer:
"Today the Neydharting moor drinking cure belongs to the most commonly used methods of healing of inflammations of the gastro-intestinal mucous membrane, ulcers of the stomach and the duodenum. By this cure the ulcer disappeared (roentgenoloically) in 90% of all cases after 3-4 weeks."

Dr. W. Thomsen, University Professor:
"... There was mentioned the nice word, "moor bouquet", In speaking of the effect of the moor on the sick body, a whole "bouquet" of healing factors is put into practice, As Mr. Stober has correctly explained to us. It concerns a large number of healing substances, which differ qualitavely. We also have the factor of the quantity.

These factors do not always exist in the same strength or quantity (not even in individual moor types and various forms of application). Therefore, we have such a large number of healing factors that it can make one dizzy, indeed. It certainly will still take a long time of research in order to determine individually these healing factors of the "moor - bouquet," as Mr Stober has told us.... We know the finest, smallest quantities often have a greater effect than the massive effect of the allopathy; and on the other hand we know that conversions of a chemical type can be delicate can be so delicate, so minimal, that grosser clinical tests simply do not respond...."

Dr. Otto Heddrich, Hannover, Germany:
"In my practice I have used your "moor gingival paste" for the treatment of chronic-recidivous *aphtae* and obtained a success as cannot be imitated by any other preparations on the market thus far...."

Dr. Walter Ehalt, University Professor, Medical Director of the Unfall Hospital, Graz, Austria:
"...that I administer your moor baths now the same as ever to my patients, and both the patients and I are very pleased with the results."

Wilhelminen Hospital, First Medical Department, Vienna, Austria; Dr. H. Siedek, University Professor, and Dr. H. Hammerl:
"...We became convinced of the favourable effects of the "drinking moor" with 300 patients within the past few weeks."

"... The moor *Schwebstoff* treatment of diseases of the gastro-intestinal tract certainly plays a highly significant role. In hyperacidic gastritis and ulcers of the stomach this favourable effect is attributed to the strongly absorbing effect of the "drinking moor." But that also spasm-eliminating factors play a role beside the inflammation inhibiting factors, is shown by the results of treatment in the case of spastic obstipations..."

Ico Salec. M.D., Zagreb (Agram), Yugoslavia:
"Neydharting moor drinking cure in gastritis, enteroptosis, dystonia -very good."

Stefan Perndl, M.D., Pfandl, near Bad Ischl, Austria:
"Have gained good results in patients with *ulcus ventriculi* by the moor drinking cure."

Karl Heinz Weber, M.D., Murau:
"...Moreover, I want to mention that essential advantages with the bathing cures can be obtained, when moor drinking cures are administered at the same time.

Karl Reinprecht, M.D., Klagenfurt, Austria:
"The mode of living of the majority of the people, their nutrition and the unnatural and irregular sleeping habits disturb the organism. The elimination of the "sludge" and poisonous matter is slowed down, and the liver is overburdened. The physician recommends the Neydharting moor drinking cure for its relief. Headaches, sleeplessness, feeling of discomfort and digestive troubles are usually quickly eliminated....Healing moor also has an antibiotic (germi cidal) effect."

General Public Hospital, First Medical Department, Klagenfurt, Austria; Director: Dr. Ignaz Kallus, Privy Councillor, Superior Medical Officer:

"...We have used the Neydharting moor *Schwebstoff* as moor bath, and we also employed the moor drinking cure. The results were very satisfactory in reference to chronic arthritis and polyarthritis as well as especially in the case of spondylarthrosis. The subjective pains greatly improved already after some baths... In the cases of ulcers of the stomach and the duodenum, in the cases of pre- and post-ulcerous gastritis and duodenitis... We have administered the drinking cure with satisfactory results.... But the value of the Neydharting moor drinking cure was shown to me in the treatment of the therapy-resistant ulcers and inflammatory processes of the mucosa, so that for these cases especially the moor drinking cure represents the therapy of choice...."

Ernst Gasporoti, M.D., Lienz:
"I recommend the Neydharting moor drinking cure for gastritis, meteorism and flatulence."

Helmuth Jesch, M.D., Gmund:
"... In the same way, excellent results were obtained by the healing moor drinking cure. I can highly recommend it for disorders of the stomach."

Dr. Franz Mitteregger, Chief Physician, Graz, Austria:
"Because of threatening *ileus* phenomena a patient had to make the decision to undergo a laparotomy because of danger to life. After a three week application of moor Schwebstoff the condition subjectively improved. The

Roentgen-control verified in a striking manner the objective improvement. After three months the patient was ready to go to work."

Siefgried Plattner, M.D., Gmund:
"Last summer I have used the drinking cure for twenty stomach ulcers and all patients were healed without operation."

Helmut Richter, M.D., Villach, Austria:
"Complete freedom from complaints were obtained after the moor drinking cure (in the cases of gastritis, ulcers of the duodenum, which did not respond to the usual conservative therapy)."

Walter Rusch, M.D., Specialist, on Skin Diseases, Bregenz, Austria:
"I confirm the excellent results of a drinking and bathing cure with Neydharting moor *Schwebstoff* with a patient, who had a generalized discharge-eczema, which was treated for 4 months with the hitherto ordinary therapies without success..."

Gangolf Sacher, M.D., Specialist, Internist, The State Administration, Sick Fund, Wolfsberg:
"I am pleased to tell you that the drinking cure with Neydharting black water has been very successful with many patients, who suffered from various digestive diseases. My observations embraced especially the chronic enterocolitis with putrefactive processes in the intestine and embraced also cholecystitis."

Wilhelm Breu, M.D., University Lecturer, Vienna, Austria:
"I have repeatedly used the drinking cure as well as the *Schwebstoff* baths in the cases of internal diseases, and obtained always best results."

Richard Bayer, M.D., University Lecturer, Graz, Autria:
"I have hitherto prescribed the Neydharting healing moor *Schwebstoff* in the treatment of chronic inflammatory gynaecological diseases as well as in selected cases of ovarian hypofunctional states (in combination with moor drinking cures). The cure was a success and encourages for further applications."

Eug. Chrobok, M.D., Medical Officer of the Government:
"Acute bilious colics responded very well to the moor drinking cures; the attacks failed to occur. The digestive tract responds well to the drinking cures; however, mild laxatives are necessary as obstipation easily takes place."

Sepp Darbringer, M.D., Physician of the State Administration for the Sick Fund:
"Besides numerous successful moor drinking cures in less severe gastritis, I have systematically treated ten cases of roentgenologically determined ulcers of the stomach and the duodenum with 3-4 bottles of this moor liquid in the past few months, and therewith improved the complaints in a short time (except one case); and finally the complaints disappeared."

Wilhelm Duscher, M.D., Scharding:
"I recommend the healing moor from Neydharting as well as drinking cures for the treatment at home."

Werner Ernst, M.D., Physician of the Sate of Administration for the Sick Fund:
" I can say that the home-treatment with Neydharting moor baths and drinking cures has turned out well, indeed, for a great number of diseases.... The drinking cure is especially suited for all chronic digestive disorders."

Dr. Marguerite Kavan:
" I use the Neydharting moor in my cosmetic department, I am of the opinion that it has the highest astringent qualities I have ever seen. It is a most active agent, which arrests discharges."

Dr. Lore Antoine, Dermatologist, Vienna, Austria:
"... that I have used Neydharting moor for cosmetic packs for a long time, and therewith I have obtained good results in healthy or seborrhoid skin."

E. Lechleitner, M.D., Pharmacologist, The Austrian Moor Research Institute:
"... We see here the eminent significance of the metabolic performance of the moor-microflora. To it, the moor owes its genesis, and by it also the majority of the pharmaco-dynamically effective groups originate, which we must require for the chemical moor effect. This concerns substances with vitamin-properties with an antibiotic effect, hormones, effective ion-exchangers, absorbents and others. It, thereby, embraces the moor-bouquet (an expression given by Otto

Stober), a great number of substances, which correctly put, grant us the permission to speak of a 'moor therapy of totality.'"

Dr. Ceria, University Professor, Dental Clinic, University of Turin, Italy:
"... Already the initial results (concerning gum-treatment) with Neydharting moor pack were encouraging, in some cases surprisingly good...."

Dr. H. di Gaspero, University Professor, Graz, Austria:
"Critical medical experiences of many years, experiences on closest combination with exact, extensive research-results permit the medical conclusion that there are no analogous therapeutic methods, i.e. no therapeutic methods of the same kind in the balmeological field of the healing art relative to the treatment with moor products."

Dr. A. Rotovic, University Professor:
"The Neydharting moor *Schwebstoff* deserves to be employed... also after bone fractures. We are of the opinion that the patient concerned may be become able-bodied sooner."

Dr. R. Pekarek, Superior Medical Officer:
"... So, we see over and over again that great successes are obtained in many persons by the means of moor *Schwebstoff* baths, where other physical methods of treatment have failed..."

Dr. W. Benade, Franzensbad, Bohemia:
"The Neydharting moor is such a well decomposed material as is very seldom found..."

Dr. H. Lachmann, Chief Physician, The Austrian Moor Research:
"... Moreover, this Neydharting bathing additive (moor *Schwebstoff*) is superior by far to all hitherto preparations of this kind because of its exclusively natural constituents."

Dr. R. Trauner, University Professor:
"We can confirm a good therapeutic effect of the mouth-wash made from the Neydharting moor..."

Women's Clinic of the University of Erlangen, School of Obstetrics, Erlangen, Bavaria, Germany;
"... in almost all cases success succeeded our expectations. Particularly in the moor *Schwebstoff* bath is clearly superior to the other baths thus frequently administered at our institute."

Dr. R. Franz, University Professor:
"... We have used the Neydharting *Schwebstoff* for inflammatory diseases of the female genitals and sterility with best results..."

Dr. F. Kazda, University Professor:
"Neydharting *Schwebstoff* for chronic joint-diseases... with very good results...."

Dr. A. Pesce, University Professor:
"... All vegative functions of the body are heightened by the Neydharting *Schwebstoff*...."

Dr. F. Schurer-Waldheim, University Professor:
"...The Neydharting *Schwebstoff* (moor suspension)

has a great number of indications in the field of surgery...."

Dr. Ignaz Kallus, Privy Councillor, Superior Medical Officer, General Public Hospital of the State of Carinthia, First Medical Department, Klagenfurt, Austria:

"...I would like to mention one more advantage of the Neydharting moor drinking cure-an advantage to which no one has referred to yet, as far as I know:

"We are all aware of the fatal role which *cholesterin* plays in heart *infarct*, and in severe vascular diseases usually culminating in death. We are now living in an 'infarct age' and an 'economic miracle age.' Critically studying the death news, I believe there are certain connections between these two things. The 'managerial' disease is no nebulous accidental disease, but rests upon hard medical facts: physic strain, plentiful nicotine from smoking, chewing or snuffing tobacco, inappropriate eating, excessive alcohol consumption, an immense number of cups of coffee, (eventually a 'blond poisoning') and especially the sittings and discussions 'till late night hours.

"Overfatigue metabolic processes are a poison for the coronary vessels, as Hitzenburger maintained several decades ago. The 'over fatigue-poisons' themselves become paralysed for the moment by caffeine, another poison, but their damage to organs continues nevertheless. In regard to this fact, it is important to point out *the only physiological opponents against the cholesterin are the pectins* found in the moor.

Dr. Kallus, speaks of various cases and problems such as ulcers, gastritis, chronic arthritis, polarritis, spondylarthrosis etc. to quote *Dr. I. Kallus, PrivyCouncillor, Superior Medical Officer, Klagenfurt, Austria:*

"... The Neydharting moor drinking cure, which I have administered to about 2,500 patients (with a success of 93%), has a full effect also without any special diet. The remarkable, amazing thing of this cure is the fact that almost every patient is without pain already, after 3 days (!), and after 4 to 6 weeks (without interruption of his professional work) he is com pletely healed..."

Up to June, 1963 Dr. Kallus has cured by the means of the Neydharting moor drink (without operation!) 93% of 4,000 patients who were sent to him for surgery.

Dr. V. Bazala, University Professor, Zagreb (Agram), Yugoslavia:

"...In this case the moor therapy acts only as a remedy, but it should also be employed prophylactically. I do not want to establish herewith a new indication or counter-indication for the moor therapy. However, because of the excellent explanation relative to the bathing reaction, it was urgent to me to prove the success of gynaecology in balmeotherapy, which undoubtedly exists and will improve, especially after we have the moor *Schwebstoff*....

"The power of nature and naturopathy will, thereby, come to full action and effect for the prosperity of suffering and working mankind. This particularly holds good for the healing moor in its quanlitatively shortened or abbreviated form as moor *Schwebstoff,* according to Otto Stober a 'moor bouquet.' Today it is the best and most successful method of treatment in the sphere of moor...."

Dr H. A. Schweigart, University Professor, Pretoria, South Africa:
"... Now I would like to say something about the drinking cure with the black moor water which may have sorptive powers in a stronger degree, as there are many unoccupied points of attachment for ions available. If the black water (*Schwarzwasser*) enters the intestinal canal, it comes in contact with the microflora of the intestinal walls. It will accept ions, sorptively bind, can absorb microbes or can extract the mineral nutrient medium from the same, especially in regard to the heavy metals occurring in traces. These effects of the moor suspensions of the moor water may be very welcomed when a *Disbakterie* exists. A black water drinking cure should be very effective in such a case..."

Rudolf Peter, M.D., D.Sc., Professor, and Vaclav Sebek, M.D., University Lecturer, Prague, Czechoslovakia:
"The experience of some generations of gynaecologists has clearly answered the question in the affirmative whether the cure treatment forms an appropriate and really significant constituent of the gynaecological treatment. Further cure successes to which we devote our constant attention, prove that healing bathing cures have not lost their significance in modern therapy, so that we have come to the conviction that the negative attitude of many an expert, even noted American specialists, is attributable to the lack of opportunity to convince themselves in practice of the effectiveness of the bathing cures...."

Dr. H. Urban, University Professor:
"...Chronic arthritis, especially spondylarthrosis of the lumbar vertebra as well as neuralgia neuritis were treated with original Neydharting moor *Schwebstoff* baths. We are very satisfied with the results obtained...."

Municipal Hospital of Berlin, Germany:
"For months we have been using original Neydharting moor Schwebstoff for complete baths and packs in the Department of Rheumatism.... We observed a favourable, intensive effect in all cases...."

Dr. I. Kallus, Superior Medical Officer and Director of the General Public Hospital of the State of Carinthia, stated with a youthful vigour at the III. International Congress for Research on Moor at Meran that he has healed many hundreds of patients (with whom all chemical preparations known at the time were tried) by administering to them a teaspoonful of Stober's Neydharting moor drink three times daily-and nothing else. Otherwise these patients would have had to submit to an operation according to general medical opinion. And with this natural method he obtained a healing result in over 93% of the cases involved so that less than 7% had to undergo the unavoidable operation. With such healing successes, which people suffering from gastric disease obtain by the Neydharting moor drinking cure, sometimes sceptics raise the question whether it is not a magical charm after all. Dr. Kallus courageously pointed out that one could call it also witchcraft in the same way if the physician requires of the patient that he may trust him. And yet we cannot speak here of a magic effect.

Dr. W. Blumencron, University Lecturer, Vienna, Austria:
"...I wish to point out that the practitioner really has something in the Neydharting moor *Schwebstoff* bath, which he can successfully employ also in the home of the patient; and this seems to me the fundamental advantage, which is far more important to the practitioner than all theoretical explanations about divergences of opinion...."

Professor Dr. Greif states: "The duodenal secretion of patients, whom we treated with the Neydharting moor drink, was investigated; and after some days an essential decrease of the pathogenic germs was ascertained. It was remarkable that the aureomycin-sensitive germs disappeared first....It showed itself that the Neydharting moor drinking cure proved very good in all gastritis, duodenities as well as in various ulcers of the stomach and the duodenum (*ulcera ventriculi et duodeni*)...

Professor S. K. Lesnoi, Moscow, Russia:
"Among the present methods of conservative treatment of inflammatory and functional gynaecological diseases, the mud therapy (treatment with moor, mud, peat), especially the balmeological one, must be regarded as a very effective therapeutic remedy...."

Dr. Max Sternad, Superior Officer of Health, President of the Upper Austrian Chamber of Medicine, Linz on the Danube, Austria:
"...I am delighted in confirming that for years I have repeatedly had the opportunity to convince myself of the extremely favourable effect of the Neydharting moor bath....The result of the cure was very good, indeed."

Professor Dr. J. Kowarschik, Privy Councillor, Vienna, Austria:

"With the introduction of the naturally pure Neydharting moor suspension (Moor-Schwebstoff) by Otto Stober, a true folk remedy has been given to the entire mankind."

Dr. Mario Kaiser, University Professor, Member of the International Medical Academy, Rome, Italy, former Director of the Hygienic Institute of the University of Vienna, Austria:

"...The reputation of the moor from Neydharting is an excellent one, both in the wide public and also in physicians' circles...."

Friedrich Fusko, M.D., Ascbach, Austria:

"I can highly recommend the Neydharting moor-cure for all rheumatic diseases as well as women's diseases and diseases of the stomach liver-tract. I have seen excellent results."

Heinz Dunkl, M.D., Salzburg, Austria:

"Some months ago I administered the Neydharting drinking cure to a female patient, 59 years of age, who had a chronic gastritis (after *ulcus duod. et. ventric.* for years). I am happy to tell you that the subjective troubles of the patient completely disappeared after completion of the cure, and they have not yet re-occurred."

Professor H.E. Stocker, M.D.:

"As director and surgeon of General Public Hospital as Scharding I can highly recommend the bathing and drinking cure of the Neydharting Spa. The drinking cure as well as the moor application have been employed at my hospital with excellent results for a long time."

Dr. Bruno Samowitsch, Ashbach:
"I certainly can recommend the Neydharting moor and drinking cures for all persons afflicted with rheumatism, and in cases of abdominal complaints in women."

Helmut Heidler, M.D., Salzburg, Austria:
"I know the Moor Spa of Neydharting and highly recommend you the baths and poultices as well as the drinking cure. It would be best to start as soon as possible."

Dr. Pec, General Physician, Vienna, Austria:
"The Neydharting drinking cure has turned out well in children with poor appetite."

Fritz Hube, M.D., Bad Lauterberg, Harz Mountains, Germany:
"...However, the use of the Neydharting moor suspension for drinking cures is completely new, especially in the case of inflammation of the digestive organs including ulcers of the stomach and intestine."

Dr. Ignaz Kallus, Privy Councillor, Superior Medical Officer, General Public Hospital of the State of Carinthia, Klagenfurt, Austria:
"The Neydharting moor drinking cure has turned out to be the most sovereign remedy in the treatment of gastroduodenal ulcers, gastritis and duodenitis. Today I can enumerate far more than four thousand cases of these diseases

which I have successfully treated therewith....To such patients I have administered five times daily small meals, and one teaspoonful of Neydharting Moor Drink from three to five times per day, one-half hour before eating."

Wolfgang Holzer, M.D., Eng.D., University Professor:
"We approved the treatment with *Schwebstoff* with scepticism at the University Clinic of Graz, but we saw that we were able to obtain good therapeutic results."

Professor MUDR. Dr.med. habil. A. Kukowka, Greiz, Thuringia, Germany:
"...I personally started employing Neydharting moor *Schwebstoff* baths on myself and on patients. Out of a Saul, I became a Paul...."

Professor Dr. Ludwig Adler, New York, N.Y., USA.:
"I deem the development of the moor treatment very important for gynaecological purposes, and I am greatly impressed by what I have seen at Neydharting."

Professor Dr. Scheminzky, Head of the Balmeological Commission of the Federal Ministry of Social Administration, Vienna, Austria:
"...The quality of the naturally moist moor earth (with black water content) of Neydharting is highly distinguished. It is among the best products on the market at the present time in Austria, if not perhaps the best."

THE FOLLOWING ARE A FEW OF THE MANY EXTRACTS FROM REPORTS RECEIVED BY AUSTRIAN MOOR U.K. FROM GRATEFUL USERS OF THE MOOR LIFE AND BEAUTY PRODUCTS.

"For years I had terrible acid indigestion. This had become so bad that I was told I was on the point of developing ulcers. I really had tried everything, including various natural treatments. My doctor had even prescribed a powerful drug, but to no avail.

Then someone recommended the Moor Drink. After two weeks the acidity and the accompanying painful throbbing in my oesophagus had vanished.

Now my digestion is back to how it was years ago. I am so thankful to the Moor. Now I can eat all those tasty things I had to avoid, without any problems."

* * * * * * * * *

"Within a few weeks of starting a course of Moor Baths, the symptoms of a hormonal imbalance that has been getting worse for two years, disappeared, even when I ate foods that has exacerbated the condition. I still can't quite believe it can be quite so simple."

* * * * * * * * *

"For the last ten years or so I have been periodically troubled with eczema on my hands which is very stubborn and can be quite distressing. I can honestly say that virtually overnight the condition showed vast improvement after starting the Moor Bath course in conjunction with the Soap, Body Cream and Cleansing Lotion.

Now after about a month of using these products, my eczema has virtually disappeared and shows no sign of returning. I would therefore strongly recommend these products for anyone with skin problems.''

* * * * * * * * *

"Since using the Moor products, I have noticed that my complexion and even the texture of my skin has improved. The Face Mask, with its unique healing properties, is much more than just a beauty product. I have found it useful for all the family to help clear up skin problems or rashes.''

* * * * * * * * *

"These products are absolutely fantastic! My skin is much softer and younger looking according to friends..."

* * * * * * * * *

"I promised when we spoke on the telephone that I would write confirming the miraculous effects of the Moor on my bladder problem. I have been suffering from incontinence for some time. After the first bottle I began to notice improvements, by the end of the course I found I was back to normal as far as my bladder was concerned.''

* * * * * * * * *

"A most interesting and appreciated side effect after starting a recent course of Moor Baths - my exceedingly painful trigeminal neuralgia appears to have been cured.''

* * * * * * * * *

"I felt I must write and tell you how much I have benefited from using the Moor Baths. After the first week I felt some relief; after completing the course I realised I had suffered no discomfort for days from the arthritis of the spine. From my experience I would recommend this treatment to any like sufferers.

"I would like to say how much better I have been since my treatment with the Moor Bath. I have suffered from rheumatoid arthritis for about eight years and had given up any hope of a cure let alone effective relief. Now I can once again walk without pain and I do all my own housework."

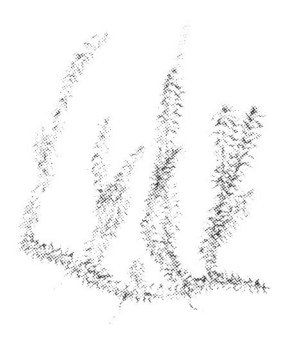

"The best service any book can render is, to impart truth, to make you think it out for yourself."

Elbert Hubbard

Cases From The Authors Practice

Female - 52 years. Suffering from extreme nervousness due to hormone changes in the menopause. Unable to sleep, hot flushes, aches and pains. Moor Baths and Moor Bouquet relieved this lady's symptoms in a matter of weeks.

Female - 16 years. Menstruation very irregular, nervous, dry skin, poor appetite, underweight. After two courses of the Bath and Bouquet, general health improved, menstruating regularly.

Female - 24 years. Had suffered from dysmenorrhoea (painful periods) for many years, also severe ovulation pains. Moor Bath and Drink produced permanent relief within six months.

Male - 8 years. Constipation and colic. Moor Drink cleared the colic within seven days. Regular stools after taking two bottles of the Drink.

Female - 32 years. Alopecia. Total loss of hair after birth of baby. Moor Drink, Shampoo and Hair Tonic resolved the problem in six months.

Baby girl - 8 months. Eczema covering whole body. After only ten days of Moor Bath, Soap and Body Cream, considerable improvement. One month later skin virtually free of eczema.

Male - 53 years. Chronic gout, knees and feet. Moor

Bath and Bouquet resolved problem within three months.

Male - 22 years. Ulcerative colitis. Severe weakness and loss of weight. Recurring boils on neck and back. Moor Bouquet produced complete healing after six to eight weeks.

Female - 56 years. Periodontal disease. Painful teeth and gums with bleeding for many years. Moor toothpaste, Mouthwash and Bouquet. General improvement after six months. Since commencing the Moor Treatment this patient had not found it necessary to visit her dental practitioner which was most unusual for her. Also, the extreme sensitivity of her gums and teeth were a thing of the past as was the bleeding.

Male - 28 years. Haemorrhoids with bleeding; chronic. Moor Bath and Bouquet cleared condition with two courses.

Female - 41 years. Recurring bouts of cystitis since the age of eighteen. Moor Bath and Bouquet for three months reduced the episodes considerably, also severity of symptoms and occurrence. After five courses of treatment this patient remained symptom free for fourteen months.

Female - 34 years. Endometriosis with much pain and swelling of the abdomen. Heavy dragging pain in lumbar region. Feeling of enervation much of the time, heavy periods. After eight months of treatment this lady lost all of the above symptoms.

Male - 47 years. Chronic acid indigestion. Suspected

ulcer, oesophagitis. Within only a few short weeks after having commenced the Moor Bouquet this man was practically free of symptoms. After four bottles his digestion was functioning well.

Female - 53 years. Gallstones. Painful gallbladder, almost daily experiencing considerable digestive discomfort with much nausea and belching. Taste of rotten eggs in mouth, tongue heavily coated. Moor Bouquet also Moor Bath as this lady suffered from various muscular aches and pains. Completely symptom free after ten weeks of treatment.

Male - 26 years. Rheumatoid arthritis of ankles, knees, wrists and fingers, night sweats, constipation, strong urine. After six weeks night sweats, constipation and strong urine were resolved. It took a further twelve weeks to produce a seventy per cent improvement in the rheumatoid arthritic condition.

Male - 68 years. Rodent ulcer - lobe of ear. Moor Body Cream and Drink. No trace except for scar tissue from previous surgery.

Male - 59 years. Varicose veins with a tendency to ulceration. Moor Bath, Bouquet and Moor Dressings on ulcers. Full course at intervals over two years produced a vast improvement. Between the courses this patient regularly dressed the ulcers with the Moor Paste and took the Bouquet once or twice daily as necessary.

The foregoing cases are only a few examples of the Moor's healing abilities. Over the years I have witnessed many other positive results from the Moor Life Treatments in cases of circulatory deficiency problems, chilblains, arthritis, candidiasis including thrush, psoriasis, all manner of endocrine related problems, impotence, liver disfunction, neuralgia, neurasthenia, auto immune diseases including M.E. herpes, simplex and zoster, glandular fever, muscle and joint injuries, burns, wounds, etc., etc.,.

With regard to the foregoing reports it has been necessary to conceal the identity of all individuals in order to preserve their privacy.

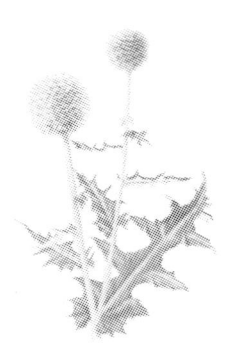

"*Nature is the means whereby the Almighty cures the ailing*"

The Neydharting Moor Clinic

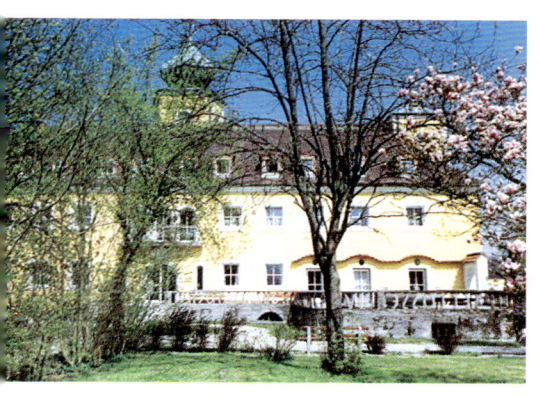

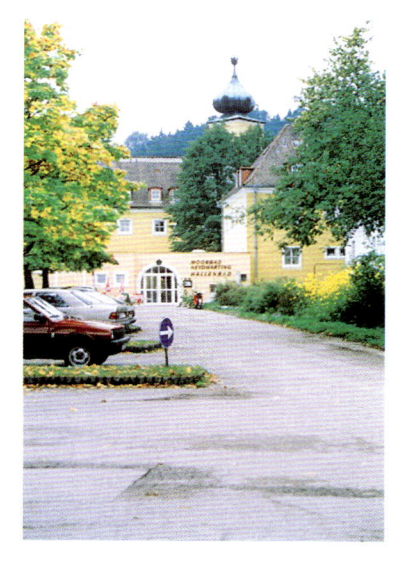

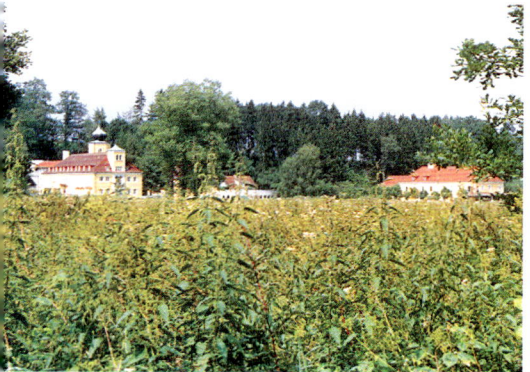

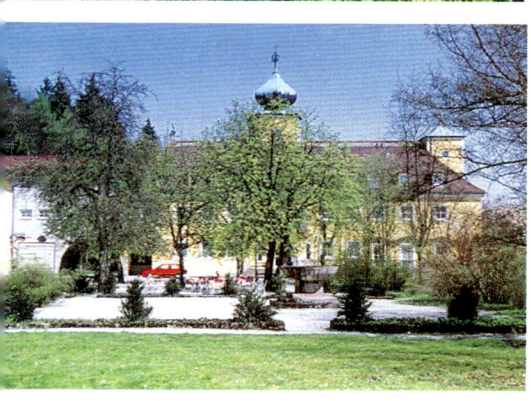

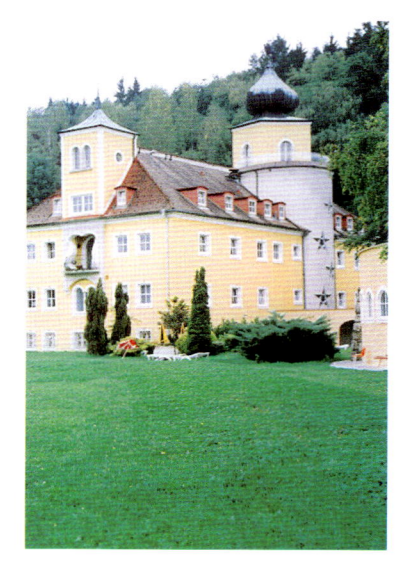

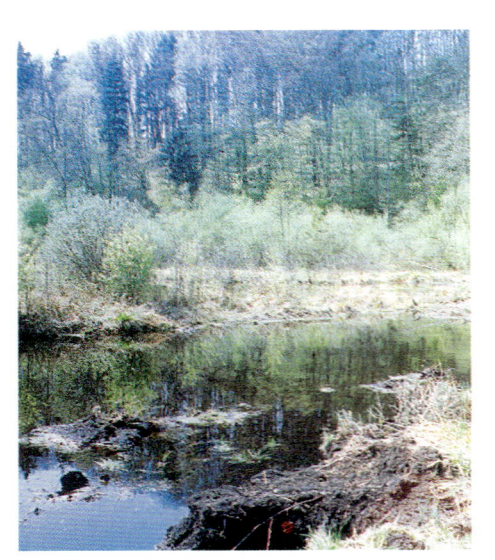

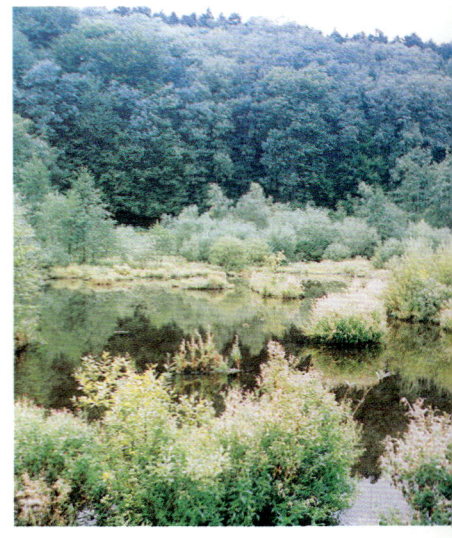

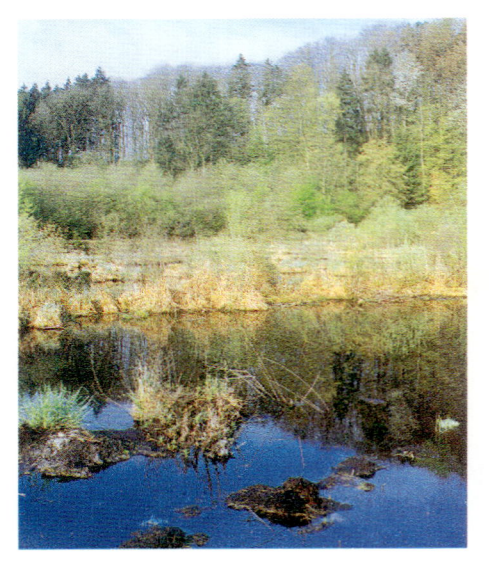

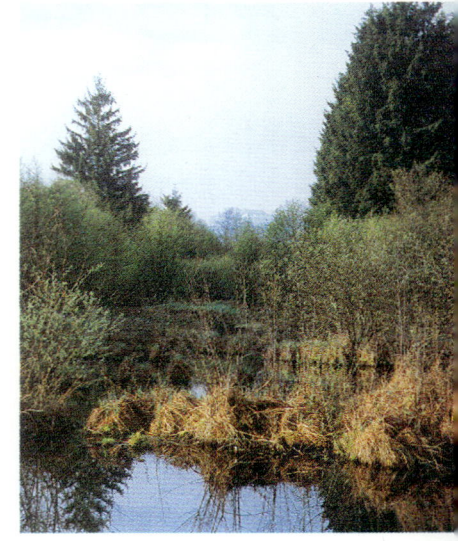

The Moor

The Moor

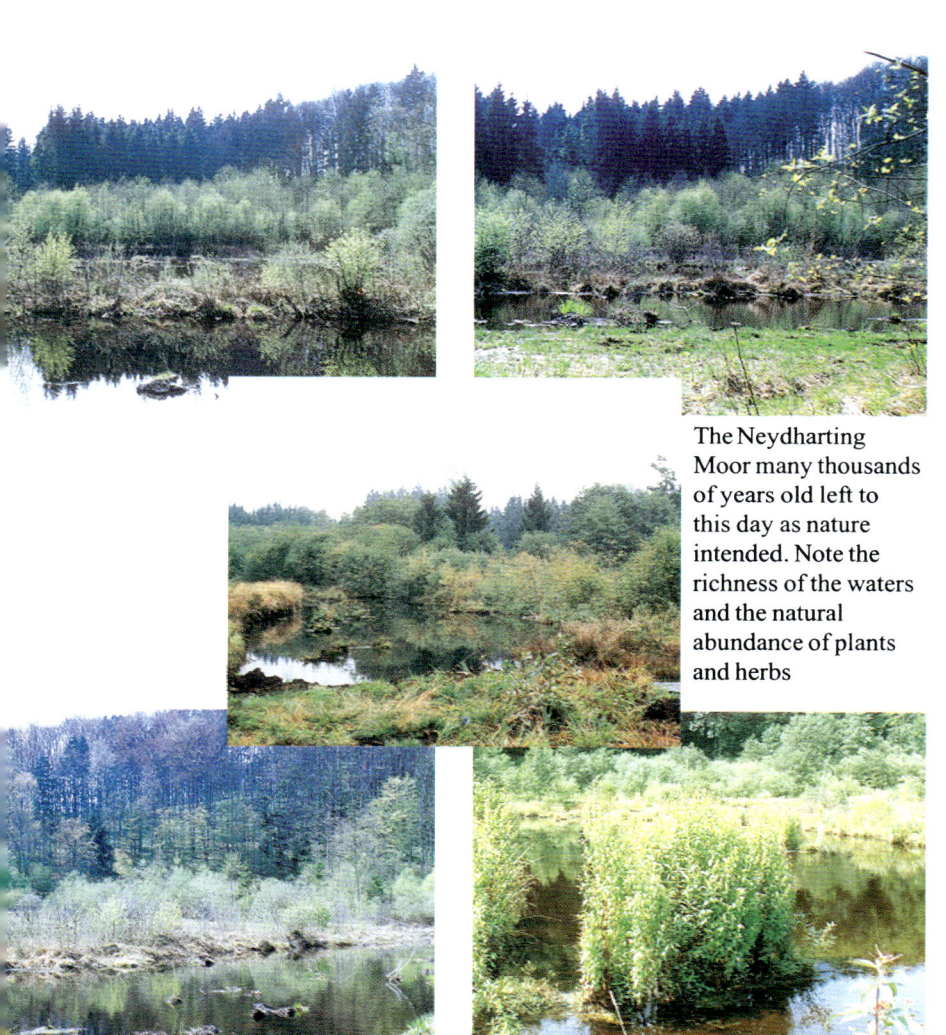

The Neydharting Moor many thousands of years old left to this day as nature intended. Note the richness of the waters and the natural abundance of plants and herbs

The Moor

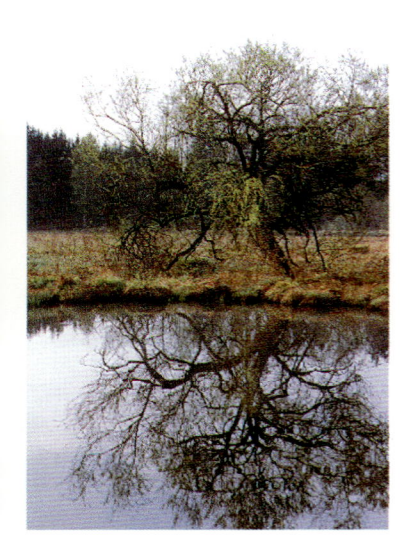

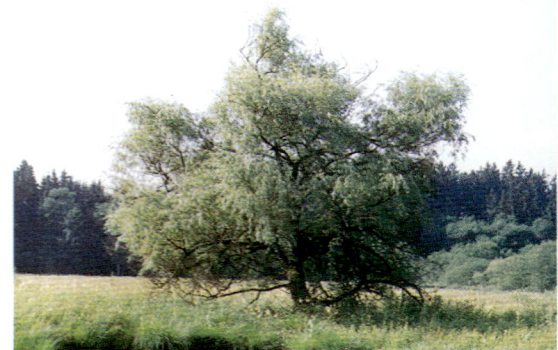

The laughing willow trees of the Moor. Note how the branches grow upwards towards the sky.

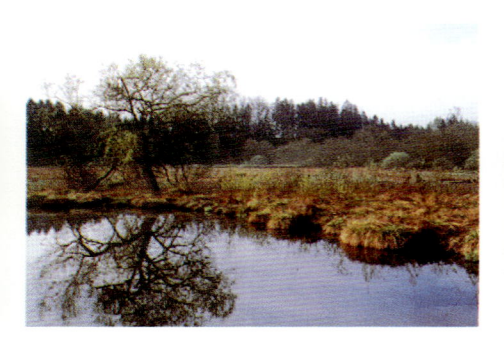

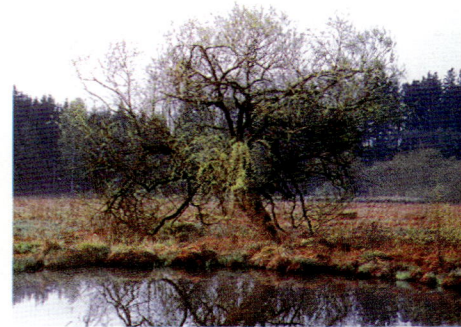

The Moor Production Centre

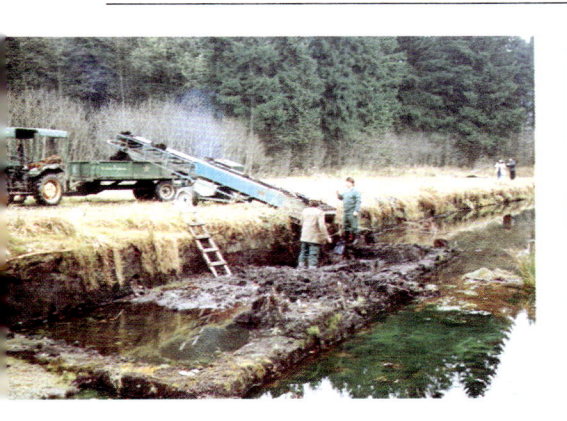

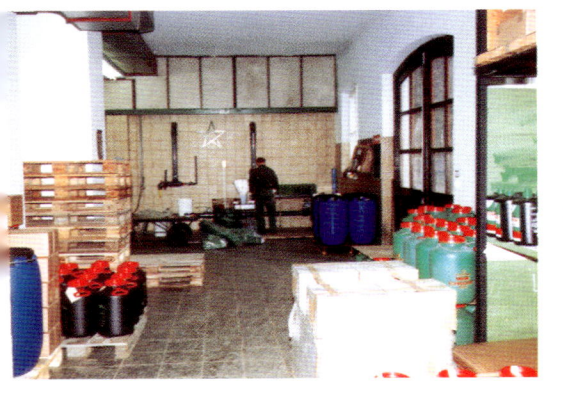

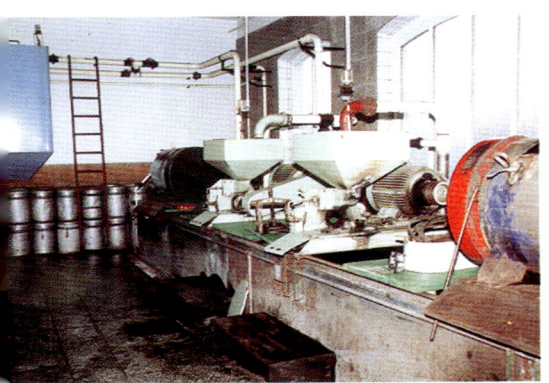

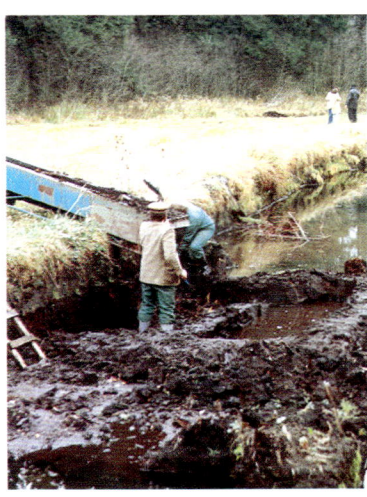

(Top left & above) Collecting the rich black mud of the Moor the production centre *(below & left)*

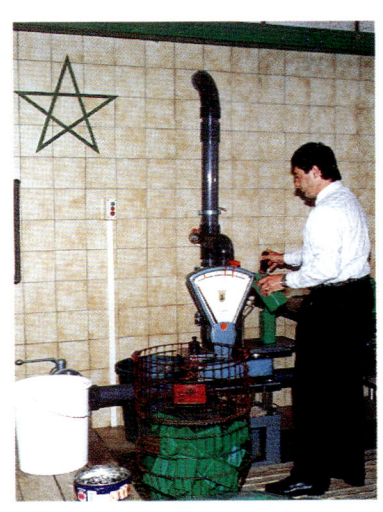

Moor Life Health & Beauty Products

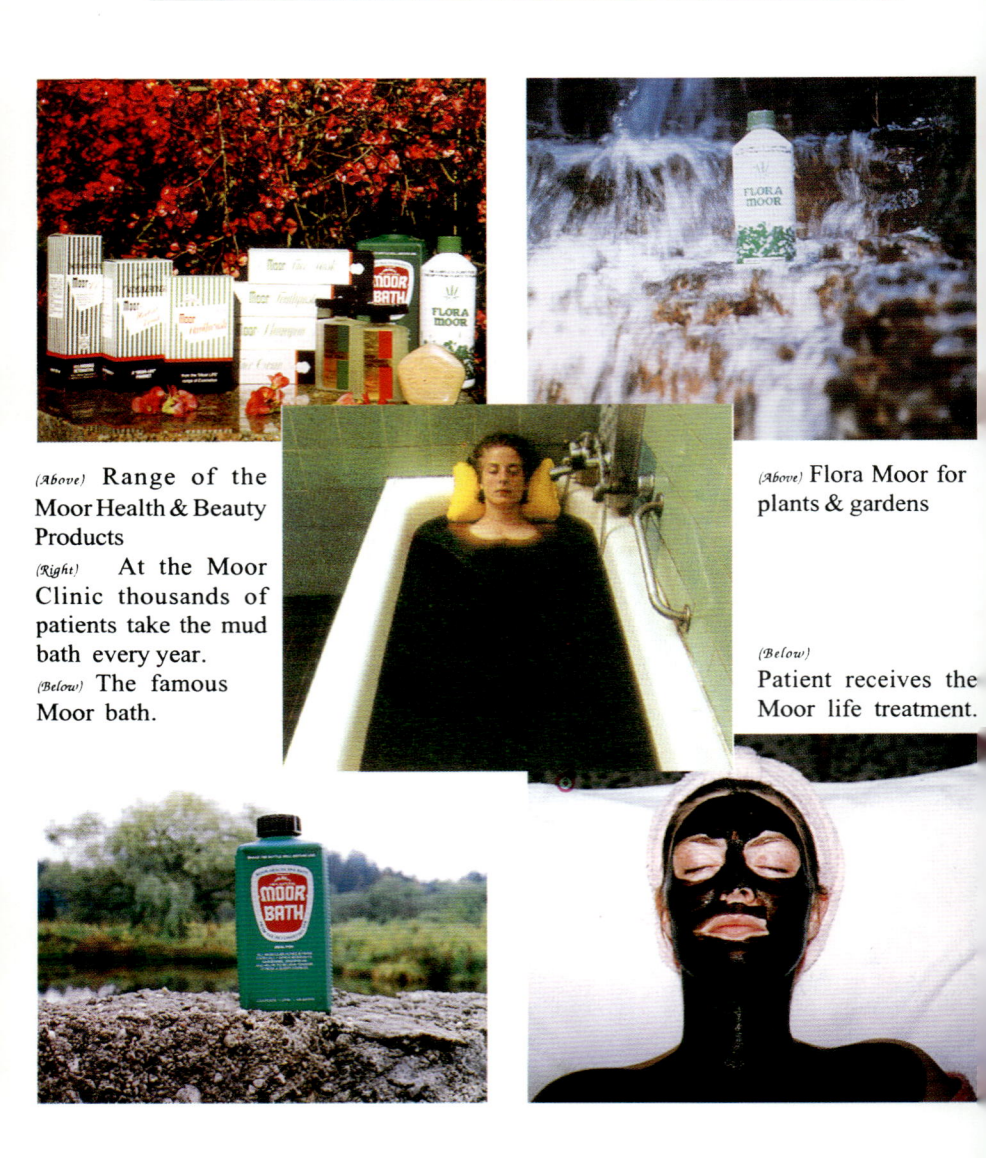

(Above) Range of the Moor Health & Beauty Products

(Right) At the Moor Clinic thousands of patients take the mud bath every year.

(Below) The famous Moor bath.

(Above) Flora Moor for plants & gardens

(Below) Patient receives the Moor life treatment.

Kirlian Photography

Please refer to page 92-93 for Nigel Garion-Hutchins report and observations on the subtle energy fields that the Moor samples clearly illustrate.

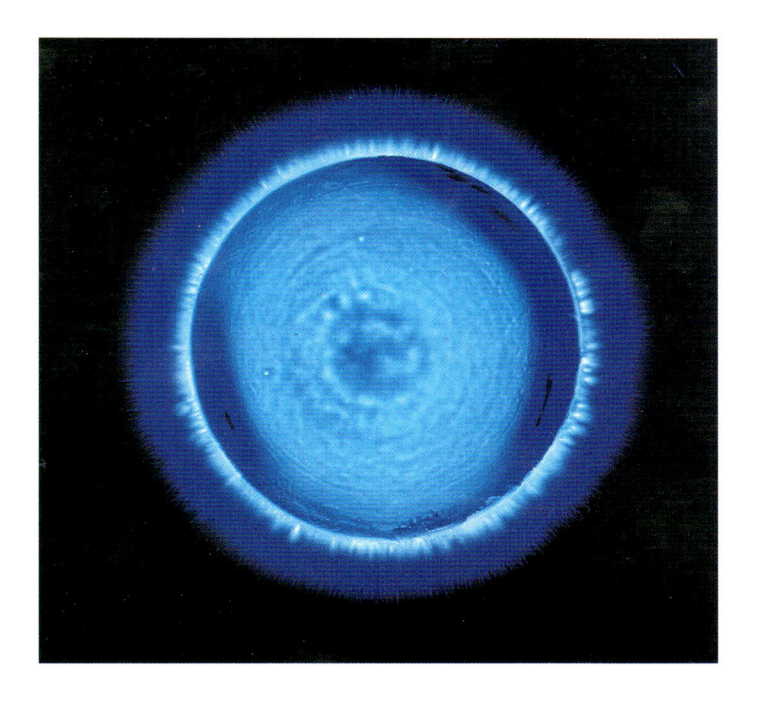

Moor Bathing Liquid
15ml in glass petrie dish.

Kirlian Photography

Please refer to page 92-93 for Nigel Garion-Hutchins report and observations on the subtle energy fields that the Moor samples clearly illustrate.

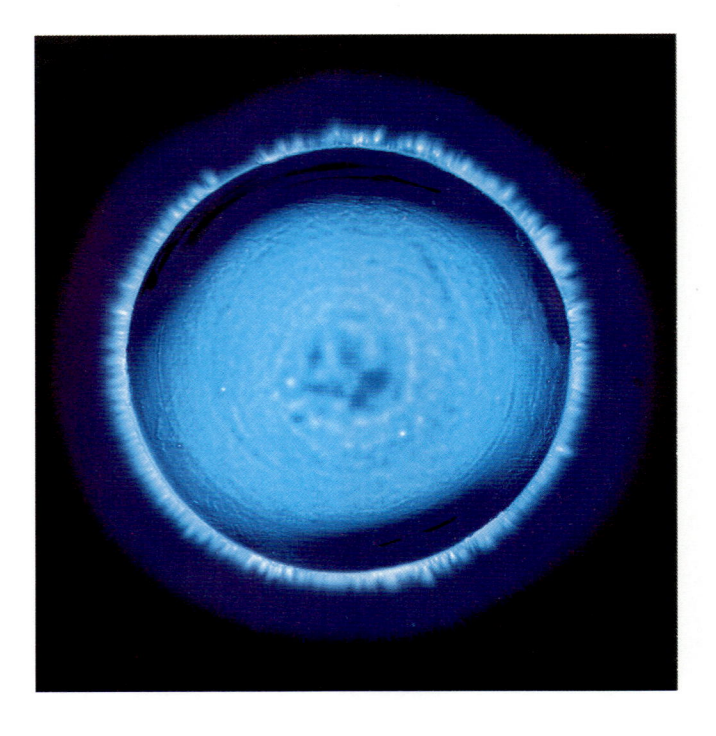

Moor Bouquet (Drink)
15ml in glass petrie dish

Kirlian Photography

Please refer to page 92-93 for Nigel Garion-Hutchins report and observations on the subtle energy fields that the Moor samples clearly illustrate.

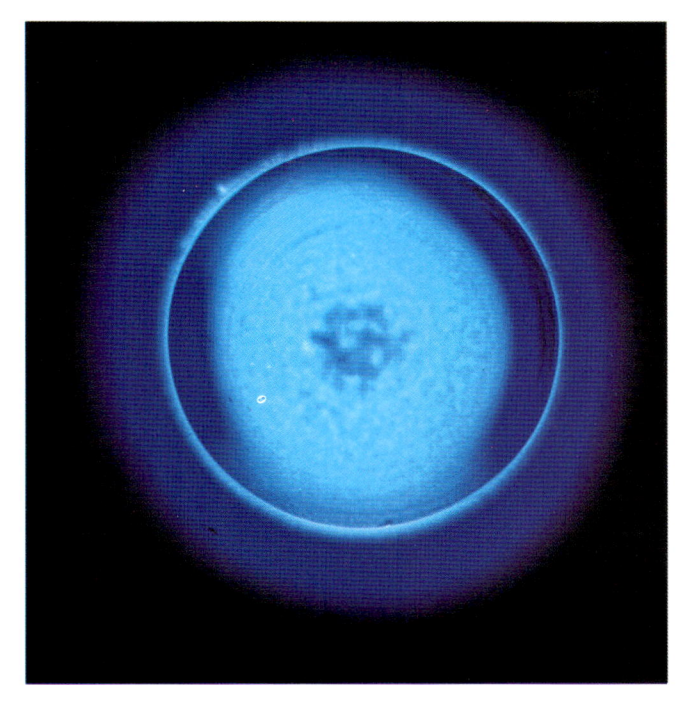

Moor Massage Oil
15ml in glass petrie dish

Kirlian Photography

Please refer to page 92-93 for Nigel Garion-Hutchins report and observations on the subtle energy fields that the Moor samples clearly illustrate.

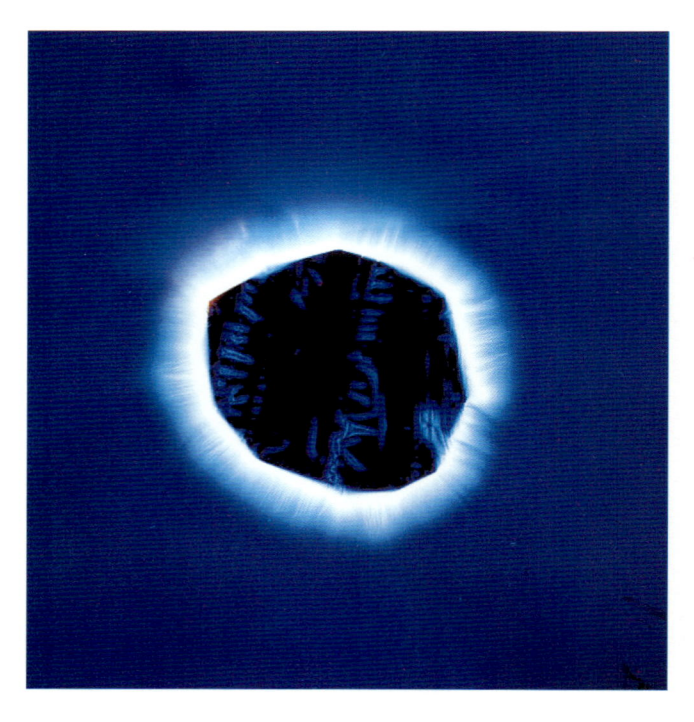

Moor Bathing Liquid
15ml in polythene container

Kirlian Photography

Please refer to page 92-93 for Nigel Garion-Hutchins report and observations on the subtle energy fields that the Moor samples clearly illustrate.

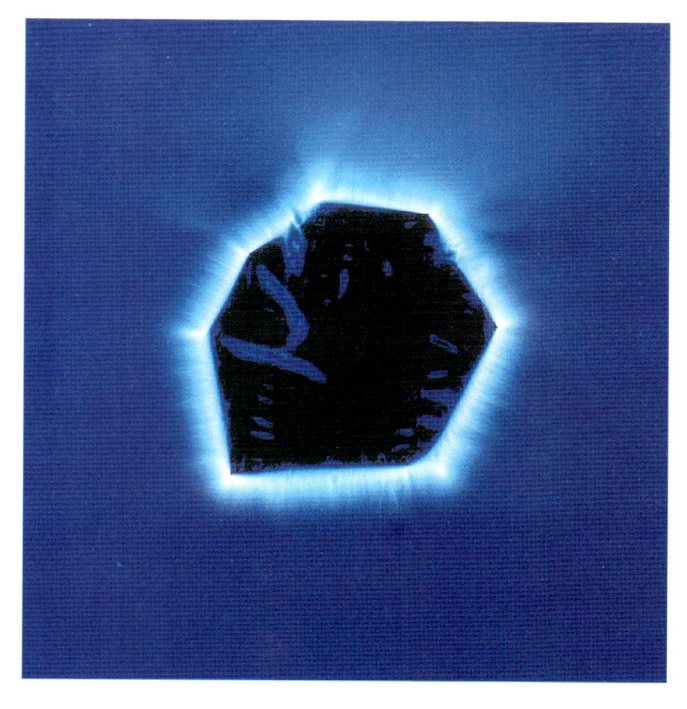

Moor Bouquet (Drink)
15ml in polythene container

Kirlian Photography

Please refer to page 92-93 for Nigel Garion-Hutchins report and observations on the subtle energy fields that the Moor samples clearly illustrate.

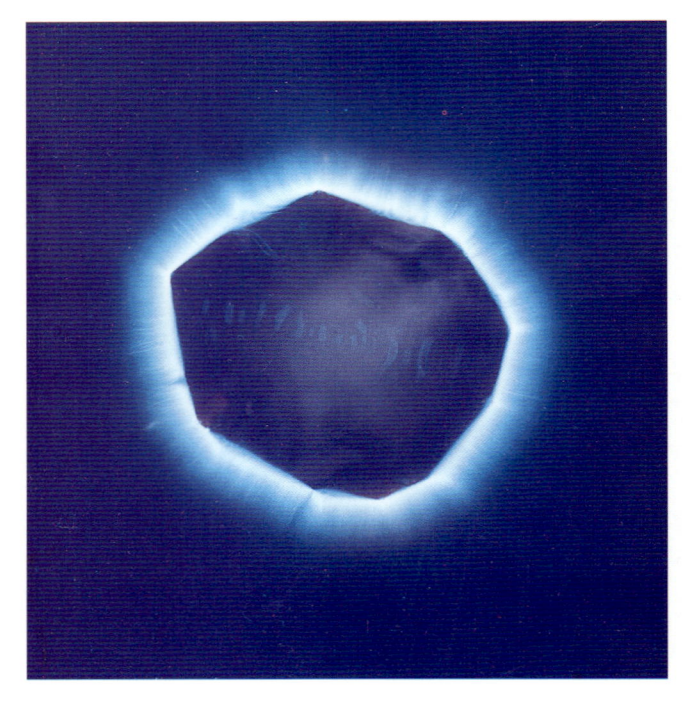

Moor Massage Oil
15ml in glass petrie dish

Healing Reactions

Some people experience soon after commencing the Moor Bath and Drink a slight worsening or exacerbation of their symptoms. This should not be taken as a negative response to the treatment, on the contrary, it is indicative of the body's innate healing reactions to the Moor's curative effects.

As the deep healing action of the Moor removes accumulations of harmful toxic materials from the organs and tissues some form of physical discomfort can occur. So as to speed up the elimination of these toxic substances I recommend increasing the fluid intake especially water, the best for this purpose is Still water on account of it's excellent flushing effects.

No matter what manifestation the healing reactions take they are necessary and favourable and should be regarded in whatever form presented an important part of the organisms self-healing efforts to illness and disease, and are not in actual fact part of the disease process. Once these healing effects pass one can confidently look forward to a grater sense of well being and health. I therefore earnestly ask the reader to most thoroughly comprehend the foregoing.

Dietetic Considerations

Although no special dietetic programme is necessary unless otherwise prescribed by your medical advisor whilst undertaking the Moor bathing and drinking course it would considerably enhance the Moors healing work if the following dietary aspects are considered.

Don't over eat, for over eating robs the brain of clear-thinking, it also makes the brain sleepy. Eat light meals, consider plenty of green vegetables, fruit, salads etc. Avoid sugar and junk foods. A natural diet helps to maintain health and fitness including mental fitness, remember certain foods especially the refined junk foods create stress within the organism.

Wrong food especially the adulterated, de-vitalised foods, stimulants such as alcohol, coffee, strong tea, salt (sodium chloride), refined sugars, flesh foods, all place considerable stress upon the adrenal glands and organs of digestion which in turn has a most damaging effect on the whole body, both on the physical and mental levels.

The following dietetic suggestions are considered well balanced. As a poor diet can create illness, so too can it be used as a means to help remedy it. Any dietary reforms attempted should be considered a lifetime habit and not just something of a temporary nature until you are well. In this way you stand a better chance of remaining healthy.

1. Select your food wisely, and masticate it well.

2. Replace all white flour and white flour products with wholemeal wheat or rye bread and flour. Replace sugar with

honey. Malt syrup, Molasses and Maple syrup can be used sparingly. Replace common salt with Bio-salt Ruthmol,or sea salt or better still eliminate salt altogether. Replace polished rice with whole grain. Replace animal fats with unrefined vegetable oil especially olive oil and use unsalted butter or cold-pressed vegetable margarine.

3. Include more fibre in the diet i.e. muesli, oats, millet, wholewheat pasta, brown rice, rye or any other wholoegrain. Increase on fresh salad vegetables, fresh and dried fruits. Vegetables should be conservatively cooked in a minimum of water or steamed. Potatoes are best cooked in their jackets.

4. Reduce considerably on all flesh foods, a vegetarian diet is considered more healthy by many scientists and members of the Medical Profession. There is irrefutable evidence proving that meat is a contributory cause of certain forms of cancer also cardio-vascular disease. Adequate protein can be obtained by combining legumes, wholegrains, rice, millet, soya, seeds such as sunflower, pumpkin, sesame, sprouted seeds, nuts, cottage cheese, yoghurt (made with proper lactbacillis culture). and free range eggs.

5. Endeavour to avoid tinned and packaged foods as they usually contain chemical flavourings, preservatives and colourings etc.

6. Do not drink with meals. Mixing food and drink delays digestion thus causing flatulence and other digestive com plaints.

7. The early morning and late evening drink should consist of spring water a little freshly squeezed lemon may be added if desirable. Quantities of spring water, herbal teas, or natural unsweetened apple, grape, orange juice may be taken at periods throughout the day

8. Endeavour to refrain except on odd occasions from coffee, cocoa, alcohol, strong tea.

9. There is a tendency to eat to much cooked food. You would therefore be well advised to increase greatly the amounts of raw fruits and vegetables. Get into the habit of eating salads all the year round.

10. Cultivate a relaxed and pleasant atmosphere at the meal table and eat only when hungry. Don't eat prior to retiring.

11. Herbs may be used to prepare cooked foods:

12. Remember the following "Let food be thy medicine and medicine thy food" - Hippocrates.

Spend some part of the day out of doors, walking sunshine is necessary to enable your body to obtain its supply of vitamin D. Fresh air is necessary for oxygenising the blood, by deeper and more vigorous breathing, thus you quicken the whole functioning of your body, speeding up the burning of your body's fuel and eliminating waste. Exercise is important as it prevents the organs and muscles from getting sluggish and flaccid and keeps them in good tone.

Muscles that are not used atrophy or run to unhealthy flesh. In walking, standing and sitting, maintain an upright posture.

There is a tendency after the age of 35 or 40 to slump at the shoulders. Immediately we do that the abdominal muscles sag and the chest cavity is compressed. If we allow that kind of posture to become habitual our whole organic function is carried on under a handicap.

It has been rightly observed that old age does not cause us to stoop, but that stooping causes old age. There is more than a grain of truth in that. Therefore cultivate the upright posture, check yourself every time you find your shoulders and your chest sagging forward and your abdomen sagging downward. In time the upright posture will become a fixed habit and you will feel younger and look younger.

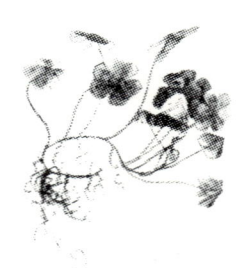

To preserve health is a moral and religious duty, for health is the basis for all social virtues. We can no longer be useful when not well.

Dr. Samuel Johnson

Authors Personal Testimony

My health began to deteriorate during the late summer of 1989. Up until this traumatic period in my life I had over the years enjoyed good health attributing this to daily early morning running of ten or more miles across the beautiful Sussex countryside which was most conducive to the release of stress caused by an exceptionally busy practice. Furthermore, over a five year period I had run in twenty five marathons usually finishing the twenty six miles in around three hours which is considered good for someone in their fifties. On one occasion I ran four marathons in one month experiencing no after effects from the effort, in a curious way I considered myself "immortal" and immune from illness.

My first awareness of anything wrong was a general and constant feeling of fatigue followed within a week or two by vague bodily aches and pains, headaches, digestive disturbances, palpitations, occasional throat infections, sore glands, uneasy and disturbed sleep and a feeling of anxiety, furthermore, around this time a series of painful tongue and mouth ulcers appeared.

I made up my mind then to undertake decisive measures in an effort to regain my previous good health by following a course of homoeopathic medications and various vitamin and mineral supplements including adherence to a strict dietetic regime. As running was out of the question; even walking short distances left me feeling wretched, I decided to increase my daily routine of hatha yoga and Tai Chi, Chi Kung excercises which I had practised in a limited and irregular manner for many years.

After twelve months of persistent and tenacious effort my health was somewhat improved. However, the general symptom pattern remained unchanged although less severe, it was then that I finally decided to undertake a course of the Moor Bath and Bouquet treatment and if necessary continue no matter how long until I felt well and symptom free. This I carried out over a period of time experiencing with each subsequent course of treatment an increased sense of health and wellbeing which has remained to this present day, although on occasions I can still experience in a much lesser and minor way, some of the previous mentioned symptoms. However, I can most definitely state I am ninety nine per cent cured.

In my own case it was not until I resorted to the deep healing powers of the Moor that I really began to recover my lost health and wellbeing which on reflection I now realise was due to a depressed auto-immune system resulting from many years of overwork both in my professional capacity as a natural medicine practitioner and my love of long distance running.

Finally, my wife and I are enthusiastic users and advocates of the Moor Life Health and Beauty treatments taking the bathing and drinking cure with regularity as a prophylaxis, furthermore, my wife carries out the Moor Life Beauty Care Routine throughout the year.

Being that the human organism contains all the elements of nature and that nature created the Moor it is therefore logical to assume that working together in perfect balance and harmony this ideal partnership must act as a powerful force against all manner of diseases.

In Perfect Harmony with Nature

The Moor's wealth of healing and therapeutic substances derived from thousands of herbs and plants in their complete totality and synergistic balance must in my opinion have a far greater and profound healing effect whether taken internally or indirectly through the skin then the single herb or combined herbal formula which may in some situations create a disturbance in the natural equilibrium within the human organism.

The Moor completely and naturally regenerates itself yearly at the rate of one millimetre. At the present rate of production and consumption scientists at the Austrian Moor Institute estimate that ample supplies should last for the next eight hundred years.

As no harmful chemical agents and herbicides have ever been used on the Neydharting Moor the natural biological balance of the local ecological system is unharmed and remains the same now as it was all those many thousands of years ago. Furthermore, no damage has occurred to the environment around the Moor, as a result, the numerous plants, fauna and wild life live in perfect balance and harmony in accordance with natures constructive laws and principles.

Moor Life, Health and Beauty products originate entirely from nature all are hand made at the Neydharting Laboratories. They are 100% natural and safe, furthermore, all the products have been given the seal of approval by the RSPCA, NAVS and BEAUTY WITHOUT CRUELTY. For over forty years Moor Life products have remained unchanged both in quality and efficacy, considering the wealth of healing substances derived from over one thousand different herbs, plants, grasses and flowers the Moor Life range of treatments must be "The Greenest Health and Beauty Products in the World". The Moor's role and wide range of therapeutic value in the restoration and maintenance of health is irrefutable. I foresee an exciting future of health and wellbeing lies ahead of us with Austrian Moor Life.

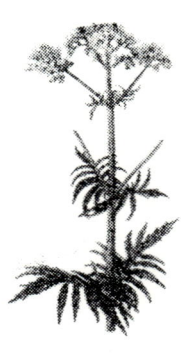

"Until man duplicates a blade of grass, Nature can laugh at his so-called scientific knowledge"

Thomas A Edison

The Moor Song

*The bountiful herbs of Neydharting Moor
give comfort and healing to those near and far.*

*O, silent and mysterious Moor with so many secrets to unfold
I thank thee for all your miracles told.*

*My heart is gladdened by the sight of majestic Neydharting
Moor so rich and black yet bright.*

*Natures healing gifts from the Moor's Bouquet
flow through those who ail that's for sure.*

*Heaven lies within nature's ancient Moor
her comforting waters every ready to heal both God's
creatures and man alike.*

*Through the healing quintessence of time-honoured Moor
may all who suffer rich and poor
find a cure for their troubles that will soon be no more.*

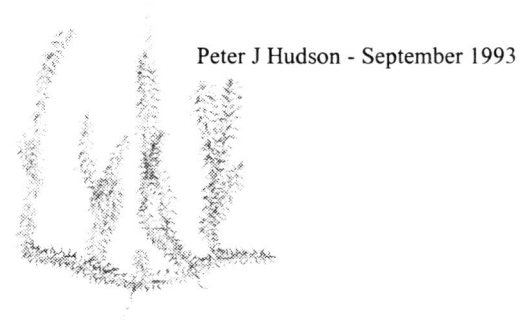

Peter J Hudson - September 1993

Conclusion

The Neydharting Moor comprehensively illuminates the basic laws and principles of nature in perfect balance and harmony. To fully understand the Moor is to understand the natural forces that engender our health and wellbeing.

This brief introduction to the Moor's miraculous healing powers has been an attempt to introduce the reader to a unique and totally holistic approach to disease in a concise and informative manner. It represents a part of the Moor's rich healing totality and tradition.

In writing this book it has been my intention to offer a basic understanding of the considerable potential and profound healing and regenerating powers of the Neydharting Moor, and to furnish practical information and helpful suggestions on the Moor's use both from a therapeutic aspect and prophylaxis.

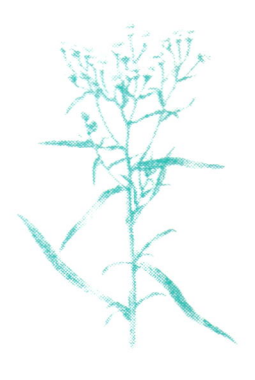

Austrian Moor UK Practitioners Association
Aims & Objectives of The Association

1. To increase awareness and acceptance by the various medical sciences and the general public of the many therapeutic applications of the Moor treatments and their wide healing potential.
2. To provide training courses and seminars in Moor Therapy for health professionals.
3. To publish papers on the application of Moor Therapy.
4. To encourage research into Moor Therapy and facilitate the dissemination of information on the subject.
5. To publish a national register of Moor Practitioners.
6. To further the application of Moor Therapy and its integration with other healing disciplines.

The Association in collaboration with Austrian Moor Life UK are currently working towards establishing the first residential Moor Clinic in this country including full clinical facilities offering the full range of traditional Moor Therapies. Considerable interest has already been shown in the furtherance of this exciting goal.

For information on courses and membership of the Austrian Moor (UK) Practitioners Association, write to the Secretary, Dolphin House, 16 Hyde Tynings Close, East bourne, East Sussex, BN20 7TQ

Austrian Moor Life UK

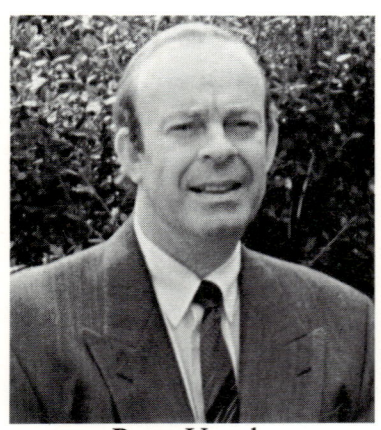

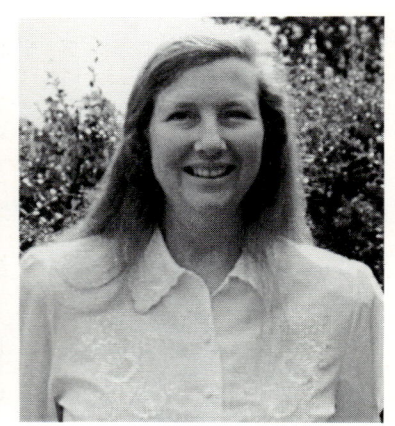

Peter Unruh
Director

Dee Unruh
Director

Information

Full details of the Austrian Moor Life Health and Beauty range can be obtained from:

Austrian Moor Products Limited
'White Ladies', Maresfield,
East Sussex. TN22 2HH.

Telephone : 0825 762658
Fax : 0825 763808

The Author

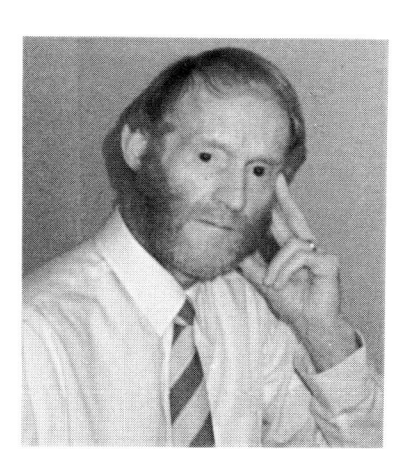

Peter Hudson has spent 35 years in the practice and study of natural medicine including Auyrvedic and Traditional Chinese medicine holding professional qualifications in naturopathy, osteopathy, herbal medicine, homoeopathy and clinical nutrition. He has run highly successful clinics in Knightsbridge, London, Kent and Sussex.

Currently Peter Hudson specialises in holistic and preventive health care as a means to achieving and maintaining health and wellbeing, he also lectures and conducts seminars and courses on holistic medicine including Tai-Chi Chi Kung and meditation and is the author of several published books and research papers.

Clinics who use the Neydharting Moor

1. **Tyringham Naturopathic Clinic** - Newport Pagnell, Bucks MK16 9ER Tel: 0908 610450

2. **Auchenkyle Health Care Ltd** - Southwoods Rd, Troon, Ayrshire Scotland Tel: 0292 311414

3. **High Glade Clinic** - 9 Upper Church Rd, St Leonards-on-sea Tel: 0424 753121

4. **Equilibrium** - Health and Beauty Complex, 150 Chiswick High Rd, London, W4 1PR Tel: 081 742 7701

5. **Ffynnonwen Natural Therapy Centre** - Llangwyryton, Dyfed SY23 4EY Tel: 09747 376

6. **Clinic of Herbal Medicine** - Acorn House, 42 Nailsworth Mills Est, George Street, Nailsworth, Glos GL6 0BT Tel: 0453 836139

7. **The Hale Clinic** - The Nutri Centre, 7 Park Crescent, London W1N 3HE Tel: 071 436 5122

8. **Natural Ways to Health** - 21 Leafield Close, St. Johns, Woking, Surrey, Tel: 0483 773958

9. **Eliz P Mallon** - 6 Edwin Street, Kinning Park, Glasgow, G51 1ND Tel: 041 427 2983

10. **Brigg Skin Surgery** - Albert Street, Brigg, Glanford, Lincs. Tel: 0652 653021

11. **Middle Piccaddilly** - Holywell, Sherborne, Dorset DT9 5LW Tel: 096 323 468

Health Hydros who use the Neydharting Moor

1. **Champneys at Stobo Castle -** Stobo Castle, Peeblesshire, Scotland EH45 8NY
Tel: 07216 249

2. **Cedar Falls Health Farm -** Bishop's Lydeard, Taunton, Somerset TA4 3HR
Tel: 0823 433233

3. **Inglewood Health Hydro -** Kintbury, Newbury, Berkshire RG15 0SW Tel: 0488 682022

4. **Grayshott Hall -** Headley Road, Grayshott, Hindhead, Surrey GU26 6JJ
Tel: 0428 604331

5. **Shrubland Health Clinic -** Coddenham, Ipswich, Suffolk, IP6 9QH Tel: 0473 830404

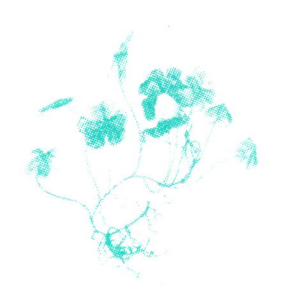

Glossary

Acidosis: Decreased alkalinity of the blood.
Adaptogen: Substances that protect the body against stress.
Adipositas: Fatness.
Alchemist: Medievil Chemistry.
Alzheimers Disease: Loss of memory for recent events and inability to store new memories.
Amino Acids: Organic elements from which proteins are constructed
Amoebiasis: Dysentry.
Anibolism: Building up of body cells.

Balneological: Therapeutic use of mineral baths.
Bio-Flavanoids: Elements required to maintain the health of the blood vessels.
Blepharitis: Inflammation of the eyelids.
Bouquet: Collection of herbs, flowers.

Candidiasis: Yeast infection.
Caries: Tooth decay.
Cellulose: Chief constituent of cell-walls of plants.
Cervicitis: Inflammation of the neck of the uterus.
Chelating: From the Greek Chelos, meaning claw.
Chloraphyll: Colouring matter of the green parts of plants.
Cholecystitis: Inflammation of the gallbladder.
Cholestrin: Waxy substance resembling fat.
Climacteric: The change of Life.

Dysmenorrhoe: Painful and difficult menstruation.
Dystocia: Difficult birth.

Effleurage: A stroking movement in massage.
Endocrine: Relating to the glandular system.
Endometriosis: Abnormal condition of the uterus..
Enzyme: Agents found in living cells that produce important chemical changes necessary for the digestion of food.

Epidermis:	*Out most part of the skin.*
Ethereal:	*Light and heavenly.*
Fatty Acids:	*Complexes of fats.*
Free Radicals:	*Highly reactive chemical elements that produce irritation of artery walls and other tissues.*
Gingival:	*The gums.*
Gutflora:	*Bacteria and other small organisms found in the intestinal tract.*
Herpes Simplex:	*Cold Sores.*
Herpes Zoster:	*Shingles.*
Holistic:	*Wholeness, wholeman, mind, body and spirit.*
Hypoplasia:	*Incomplete or arrested development of an organ or part.*
Infarct:	*Area of dead tissue frequently occurs in coronary thrombosis.*
Innate:	*Inborn.*
Ions:	*Electrically charged particles.*
Ion-Exchanging:	*Reversible chemical reaction between solids and solutions.*
Irritable Bowel Syndrome:	*Over reaction of the colon to various stimuli.*
Leucorrhea:	*Whitish discharge from the vagina.*
Leucocytes:	*White blood cells.*
Lymph:	*Colourless fluid containing white blood cells.*
Metabolism:	*Physical and chemical changes.*
Meteorism:	*Distension of stomach or intestines with gas.*
Molecular:	*Smallest particle.*
Myalgia:	*Muscular pain.*
Neurasthenia:	*Depletion of the nervous system.*
Obstipation:	*Constipation.*
Oestrogen:	*Female hormones.*

Pathogenic:	Capacity to produce disease.
Pectins:	Geletinous substances found in berries and fruits.
Pelloids:	Therapeutic substance looks like mud which is found in nature, can be organic, inorganic or both.
pH Factor:	Scale of the acidity and alkalinity factors.
Periodontal:	Inflammation of the membranes that cover the roots of the teeth.
Peristalsis:	Wavelike movements of constriction or relaxation.
Petrissage:	Kneading, rolling and picking up of muscles in massage.
Phlebitis:	Inflammation of walls of vein.
Polyarthritis:	Rheumatic - arthritic disease.
Progestrone:	Female hormone.
Prophylactic:	Prevent disease.
Prophlaxis:	Preventative treatment against disease.
Prostatitis:	Inflammation of the prostate.
Pyorrhoea:	Inflammation and gradual destruction of supporting tissues of the teeth.
Quintessence:	Purest form.
Quintuple:	Five fold.
Rodent ulcer:	Form of skin cancer
Seborrhoid:	Appertaining to the sebaceous glands of the skin.
Schwebstoff:	Held in suspension.
Spondylarthrosis:	Inflammation of the vertebrae.
Trigeminal Neuralgia:	Pain along the course of the 5th cranial nerve of the face.
Toxin:	Organic poison produced in living or dead organisms.
Vital Force:	Subtle, vital energy.

References:

Healing Earth Moor *Wolfgang Paul D.Sc.*

Guide to Optimal Health *Harold Elrick, M.D.*

James Crake, Ph.D., *Sam Clarke, M.S.*

Why Die Young

Life Extension and Rejuvenation

The Natural Way *Peter J. Hudson N.D.,D.O.*

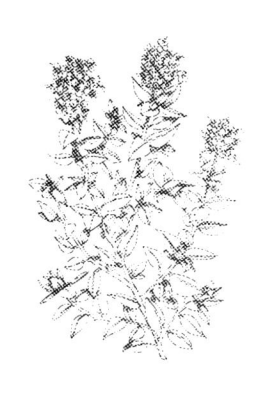

Index

A

Abdomen	31,60
Abrasions	44
Absorbent	15,104
Accidents	14,27,55
Aches and Pains	30,44,63,66,121,141
Achilles tendon	66
Acid	47,49,57,79
Acidosis	47
Acne	15,44
Acupuncture	77
Adaptogens	22
Adler, Ludwig Proffessor, Dr	114
Adulterated	47,137
Ageing	51,56,57
Albumin	28
Alchemist	1
Alkaline	45,47,48
Alopecia	119
Aluminium	36
Alzheimers disease	37
American specialists	109
Animals	1,5,41,55,56,83,84,87
Antibiotics	4,22,26,37,61,69,83,100,104
Appendicitis	68
Arm Bath	33
Aromatherapy	77
Arterial	37,73
Arth, Joseph, Dr	84
Arthritic	28
Arthritis	15,27,86,108,110,116,122
Asthma	68
Astringent	15,104
Athletes foot	15
Atoms	49
Auto-immune	122,142
Austria	2,27,59,83,86,95,99-114
Government	5,25
State	39
Moor Research Institute	3,35,38,85,88,104,143
Austrian Moor (UK) Practitioners Association	147

B

Bacteria	37

Balneological	105,108,111,114
Baltz, Edward, Dr	56
Bath	22,27,34,38,48,52,61,63,74,96,100,101,104, 110,111,115,116,119,120,142
Bayer Richard Dr.	103
Bazala. V. Dr.	108
Beauty	41,42,51,52,142,144
Beautiful	59
Bees	84
Benade, W. Dr.	105
Bible	1
Biological	2,4,26,51,143
Bio-organisms	60
Bircher, Benner Dr.	37
Birds	5
Bites	44,85
Bladder	15,32,34,38,68,116
Bloodstream	28,60
Blood vessels	27,32,76
Blumencron, W. Dr.	111
Bones	65
Bountiful	52
Bouquet (Herbal Drink)	34-39,48,59-61,63,70,72,80, 84,92,98104,109,119-121,135,142
Bowels	68,70
Breasts	31,60,62
Breu, Wilhelm, Dr.	103
British Isles	55
Bruising	65,74
Brushing Skin	30,31,52
Burghard, Breitner, Proffessor, Dr.	95
Burns	15,44,122
C	
Cadmium	36
Cancer	37,68,138
Candidiasis	122
Capillaries	28
Cardo-Vascular	37,138
Caries	46
Carrel, Alexis, Dr.	57
Cathartics	68
Catarrh	98
Cat	1,56
Cells	22
Cellulose	4
Celts	1

Ceria, Professor, Dr.	105
Cervicitis	61
Chelating	36
Chemical	28,41
Chernobyl	4
Childbirth	60
Chiropody	77
Chitil, W. Dr.	96
Cholecystitis	102
Cholestrin	107
Cholesterol	38
Chrobok, Eug. Professor	103
Circulation	15,28,32,33,45,59,67,68,73,122
Cleansing	47
Climacteric	15
Colic	16,119
Coliform Bacteria	37
Colitis	15,36,68,120
Colon	48,67-70,72
Colonic Irrigation	72
Compresses	30,65,86
Constipation	17,48,59,61,68,69,71,103,119,121
Cortisone	28
Cows	84
Cradle Cap	61
Cystitis	34,120

D

Dandruff	45
Darbringer, S.Professor, Dr.	103
Dead	5,21,31,55
Death	47
Decomposition	21
Degenerative	16
Dental	46,53,79,81,105,120
Depression	63
De-toxifying	49
Diarrhoea	61
Dietic	137,141
Diverticulitis	68
Douche	61
Drink (Herbal Bouquet)	22,27,34,48,98-100,104,108,119
Duodenal	16,36,98,101-103
Duodenitis	16,98,113
Dusher,Wilhelm,Professor,Dr.	104
Dysmenorrhoea	119
Dystonia	100

E
Ears	37
Ecological	131
Eczema	44,61,102,115,119
Effleurage	75,76
Ehalt, Walter Dr.	99
Electro-Magnetic	82-91
Elixir	55,57
Endometriosis	120
Endocrine	49,97,122
Endo Cervicitis	61
Endometritis	16
Enema	68,69
Energy	22,52
English	48
Enterocolitis	16,102
Enzymes	69
Epidermis	28
Ethereal	5
Eye	44

F
Faecal	67
Father of all healing	73
Fatigue	141
Fatty Acids	27
Female	27,34,38,68,96,106
Fertility	85
Fever	74
Fish	5
Finland	86
Flatulence	101
Flora	25,35,37,38,69
Flora Moor	87-89
Foals	85
Folklore	21
Footbath	30,32,33,82
Foot and Mouth	84
Forage Moor	83,85-87
Fractures	65,66,74
France	2
Franz. R. Professor, Dr.	106
Frigidity	34
Frogs	5
Fruit	5,88

Fusko, Fredrich, Dr.	112

G
Gallbladder	16,38,121
Gardening	66,83,87
Garion-Hutchings, Nigel	92
Gasporiti, Ernst Dr.	101
Gastritis	16,36,98,100-103,108,111-113
Gastro-Intestinal	34,36-38,98,100
Geological	2,4
Germany	2,86,95,99,106,110
Glandular Fever	122
God	15,22
Golden Key	51
Gout	16,119
Greif,Stefan. Professor Dr.	98,111
Gums	46,52,105
Gynaecological	16,27,28,97,103,108,109,111,114
Gynaecologists	59,109

H
Haemorroids	34,59,68,120
Hair	45,52,63,79,81
Hand Bath	30
Harvest Moor	83,84,87
Hatha Yoga	141
Headaches	68,100,141
Heart	33,107
Hedgeroww	42
Heddrich, Otto Dr.	99
Heinrich, di Gaspero Professor Dr.	97
Healing	23,27,29,30,32,35,44,46,51,58,61, 66,74,77,87,98,105,135,137,146
Herpes	122
High Blood Pressure	30,68
Hip Bathing	30,33
Hippocrates	73,127
Holistic	22,32,51,61,146
Holzer, Wolfgang Professor	114
Homoeopathic	93,141
Honey Bees	84
Hormonal	15,21,27,49,59,96
Hormones	4,27,29,38,62,63,97,104,119
Horses	56,83,85,86
Hot Flushes	63,119
Hube, Fritz Dr.	113
Hungary	86
Hygienic	34,38,53,81
Hypoplasia	96,97

Immortal	*57,141,*
Immune	*28,141*
Impotence	*34,122*
Incontinence	*116*
Indigestion	*59*
Infertility	*16,60*
Inflammation	*15,16,28,35,38*
Injuries	*21,27,63*
Inherent	*22*
Innate	*52,85*
Interlect	*56*
International Association for Moor Research	*3,28*
International Scientific Congresses	*15*
Intestinal	*35,37,38,70,86*
Inorganic	*21*
Insomnia	*28,63*
Intestines	*32,34*
Ion-Exchanging	*15,27,104*
Irritable Bowel Syndrome	*36*
Italy	*2,85,87,105,68,100,141*

J

Jesch, Helmuth, Dr.	*101*
Joints	*27,28,38*
Jesephine	*1*

K

Kaiser, Mario, Dr.	*112*
Kaiser, Professor Dr.	*95*
Kavan, Marguerite Dr.	*104*
Kasda, F. Professor. Dr.	*106*
Kallus, Ignas Dr.	*36,98,101,107,108,110,113*
Kidneys	*16,32,34,38,59,68,79*
Kirlian Photography	*91-93*
Klare, V. Dr.	*96*
Kostner, M. Dr.	*86*
Kotschau, Professor, Dr.	*95*
Konarschik, J. Professor. Dr.	*28,95,96,112*

L

Lachmann, H. Dr.	*106*
Lactation	*60*

Lane, Sir William Arbothnot	48
Laughing Willows	4
Laxatives	68.70.,103
Lead	36
lechleitner, E. Dr.	104
Lesnoi S. Professor	111
Lethergy	63
Leucorrhoea	34,61
Life Span	55
Ligaments	65
Liver	16,38,68,100,112,122
Living Gift of Nature	4,41
Louis XIV	1
Lumbar Region	16,110,120
Lymph	31,33,73,80

M

Magical Secrets	51
Mammary Glands	38
Manipulative	74,77
Manual Workers	66
Marrathon	66,141
9Massage	45,65,73,77
Mastitis	60,84
Meadow	42
M.E.	122
Medical Insurance	2
Menopause	16,27,34,38,62,63,119
Menstrual	16,62
Menstruation	62,74,119
Mercury	36
Metabolic	16,28,60,104,10p7
Meteorism	101
Micro Elements	21
Milk Production	84
Minerals	4,21,833,141
Miracles	22
Mitteregger, Franz Dr.	101
Molecular	4
MOOR LIFE	
Bath	52,53,61,63,65,66,92,115,119,120 135,137,142
Body Cream	33,44,60,61,63,66,82,115,119,120
Body Lotion	45
Bouquet	52,53,59,60,61,63,70,72,80,92,98 99,104,109,119,121,135,137,14277
Breastcare	52,53,60,62

    Cleansing/Toning
    Lotion   42,44,52,115
    Day Cream/Moisturiser 44,52
    Face Cream   43,44,52,53,62
    Face Mask   42-44,52,62,116
    Hair Tonic   45,52,80,119
    Massage Oil   33,45,65,66,73,74,76,77,92
    Mouthwash   46,52,81
    Shampoo   45,52,53,61.80,119
    Soap   42,43,52,60,74,82,115
    Toothpaste   46,52,53,81,120
Morning Sickness   59
Mucous membrane   34
Muscles   27,32,38,60,65,71,7l3
Myositis   86
Myalgia   16

N
Napoleon   1
Nappy Rash   44
National   1
Naturopathy   108
Neurasthenia   122
Neuorological   37
Nervous System   28,32,38,73,82
Neuralgia   16,110,122
Neuritis   16,110
Newts   5
Nicotine   107
Nipples   60
Nosema   84
Nutrition   48,57

O
Oat Seedlings   88
Obesity   28
Oesophagus   115,121
Oestrogen   29
Organic   2,3,21,23,26,88,91,128
Osteopathic   74,77
Ovaries   16,29,103
Ovulation   119
Oxygen   3,65

P
Palpitations   141
Pancreas   38

Paracelsus	*1*
Pathogenic	*69,86,111*
Paul, Wolfgang Dr.	*7,38*
Pectins	*36,38,107*
Pekarek R. Dr.	*105*
Pelliods	*2*
Periodontal	*81,120*
Peristalsis	*69,71*
Pesce A. Professor Dr.	*106*
Peter Rudolph Professor Dr.	*109*
Petrissage	*75,76*
Pets	*83,89*
Pharmaco-Dynamically	*104*
pH	*41,46*
Phlebitis	*16,74*
Physiology	*70,82,91,107*
Piles	*16*
Plaque	*81*
Platner S. Dr.	*102*
Poison	*1,35,67,69,107*
Poland	*84,87*
Polyarthritis	*108*
Ponies	*85*
Pregnancy	*59,74*
Progestrone	*29*
Prophylactic	*38,48,84,85*
Prophylaxis	*142,146*
Prostate	*27,38,68*
Prostatitis	*16,34*
Pruritis	*34*
Psoriasis	*16,122*
Psychological	*72*
Psychotherapy	*73*
Psycho-Physiological	*49*
Putrefactive	*3,102*

Q
Quinta Essentia	*1,21*
Quintessence	*22*
Quintuple	*15*

R
Radio Active	*4*
Radiations	*51*
Reflexology	*32,77*
Reinprech T. Karl Dr.	*100*

Rejuvenate	*34,49*
Reproductive	*38*
Rheumatic	*17,28,44,96,97,110,112,113*
Rheumatoid Arthritis	*17,121*
Richter, Helmut Dr.	*102*
Rockerfeller Institute USA	*57*
Roentgen	*102,103*
Rotovic A. Professor Dr.	*105*
Royal Society Great Britain	*71*
Rusch Walter Dr.	*102*

S

Sacher Gangorf Dr.	*102*
Salec Ico. Dr.	*100*
Saltzburgh	*1,113*
Salve	*42,44*
Scalp	*45,79*
Scar Tissue	*17,62,74*
Scheminzky, Professor Dr	*114*
Schweigart H. Professor Dr	*109*
Sciatica	*17*
Seborrhoid	*104*
Self-Regeneration	*22*
Senze A. Professor	*84*
Sensual	*46*
Seppia G. Del Dr.	*85*
Sexual	*34*
Siedek H. Professor Dr.	*99*
Silbert P. Dr.	*86*
Sitz Bath	*30,33*
Skin	*17,28,29,31,37,42,46,51,52,60,63,116*
Sleep	*32,119*
Sleeplessness	*59,68,100*
Sore Throats	*46*
Soul	*41*
South Africa	*109*
Spiritual	*92*
Spondyl-Arthrosis	*17,101,108,110*
Sportsmen and Women	*45*
Sterility	*17.97,106*
Stings	*44*
Stober, Otto, Professor	*2,3,22,27,36,41,70,104,105,108,110,112*
Stockholm	*66*
Stocker H. Professor Dr.	*112*
Stomach	*32,34,36,61,74,86,98,101,102,112,113*
Stretch marks	*44,60,62*
Stress	*22,65,73*
Subtle	*22,82,91*
Sulfonamides	*37*
Sunburn	*44*
Surgery	*36,107,108*
Sussex	*141*
Switzerland	*2,37*

T

Tae Chi Chi Kung	41
Teeth	46,52,81
Tendons	65,86
Thermal	28
Therapeutic	5,15,23,27,28,36,73,105,106,111,114,144
Thomsen. W. Professor Dr.	98
Thrush	34,61,122
Thyroid	80
Toxin	47,49,57,71,79
Toxic	36,37,68,88,89,135
Traumatic	27
Trauner, R. Dr.	106
Trigeminal Neuralgia	116
Tumours	74

U

Ulcers	46,98,101-103,108,113,121
Universal Moor Research	5
United Kingdom	27,87
Urban, H.. Dr.	110
Urinary	37,63
Uterine	17
Uterus	60

V

Vaginal	17,37,61,63
Vaginitis	17,34,61
Varicose Veins	28,60,68,74,121
Vegetative	28,106
Venous	73
Veterinary	83,84
Vienna	86,95,96,113
Viral	84
Vital Force	22,51,55,57,88
Vitality	41,51
Vitamins	4,21,27,83,104,127,141
Volitile Oils	38

W

Waldheim, Shurer. F. Dr.	106
Wildlife	89
Willow Trees	4
Wind	61
World	3

Y

Youth	51,55
Yugoslavia	100,108

Z

Zaribricky, F. Professor	15

Notes